I Survived the Attack of the Killer Boobie!

Jamie C. Batson

I Survived the Attack of the Killer Boobie!

ISBN: 1492746096
ISBN-13: 978-1492746096

DEDICATION

This book is dedicated to my wonderful husband Bruce, my beautiful daughter Zoe, and the multitude of friends and family who supported me through this long journey. (Zach, Adam, Angie, Ben, and Sarah, you are included. You were just out on your own when the journey began!)

I Survived the Attack of the Killer Boobie!

CONTENTS

I Survived the Attack of the Killer Boobie!

ACKNOWLEDGMENTS

Many heartfelt thanks to the many doctors and nurses who worked so hard to help me beat cancer. May God bless them all!

My utmost gratitude to Harrison Acosta whose faith in my writing and request to use it for his UIL competition spurred me into completing this book.

Thanks also go to my youngest sister, Courtney Headley for the cover art. Great job, Sis!

Special thanks go to my mother, Marsha Craig, who offered to help with the editing. Even though I did not take you up on your offer, the fact that you made the offer was noted and appreciated!

Editing assistance was provided by Toya Woods, Chris West, Zoe Batson, Bruce Batson, and Donna Trout. Your input has been invaluable in preparing this book for publication and putting the final "tweaks" on it! This work is so much better with your assistance than I ever possibly could have made it on my own!

Thanks also go to my dear friend and colleague, Susan Spring, who took one look and helped me to see some of the more glaring errors in my early work on the story.

I Survived the Attack of the Killer Boobie!

1
7-6-11 ACCOUNTABILITY/SETBACKS

Today was the first day this month I was able to get out and walk. As with most goals in life, I have been facing a setback. It is a physical condition that I can overcome with considerable time and probably medication. I have a 'breast mouse'. Right now, all we know is that I have one. We don't yet know what the nature of the 'beastie' may be, but hope to know more today after an ultrasound is performed on it.

When I got up this morning, I took the pain medication I received from the doctor yesterday, and then had a wonderful surprise . . . my daughter got out of bed and walked with me! It was a very pleasant morning, and she provided excellent company as we walked along. The pedometer read 2.88 miles when we made it back home.

There is truly something satisfying about walking with your daughter and just talking about nothing and everything. It made the journey so much more special for me.

In spite of the setback, I have maintained my loss of 20.5 total body inches. I suspect that once we get the swelling down from where things showed up on Friday night, it will be much better.

2
BIGGER SETBACK . . . CONSIDER IT A CHALLENGE

Last week was interesting. I only managed to walk on two days. I spent the rest of my time in doctor's offices and on the road between doctor's offices. The week ended in a surprise surgery.

It all started . . . or I at least became aware that it had started . . . on the last Saturday in June. We had gone to El Paso for the weekend. On Saturday evening, I noticed a place in my left breast that felt 'different' to me. I asked my husband, Bruce, when we went to bed if it felt like a lump to him. I guided his hand to what I thought felt different. After a few moments, he told me that he wasn't sure, but it just felt like a rib to him.

One week later, at the start of the Independence Day weekend, I suppose I should say just after midnight on July 2, I woke from a deep sleep, screaming in pain. (I have never been a screamer.) It felt like someone was pouring molten lava into my breast in the area that I had been concerned about just one week before. I reached to rub it and found a soft knot the size of a goose-egg. My cry had awakened Bruce too, and as couples who have long years together and are comfortable with helping each other do, he tenderly reached to try and rub out the knot. After about 30 minutes, he had it down to a more manageable size, but quit rubbing when he hit a spot that caused that lava like feeling to once again surge forth.

I frantically headed to the bathroom to try and express out the pain. (When I had been breastfeeding and would have milk to feed the nations, I often had to do this to get to a more comfortable state.) Unfortunately, there was no change in my pain level from doing this, and hindsight makes me wonder if it might have possibly caused the extreme speed with which events began to unfold later.

Being a holiday weekend, I knew that I would not be able to see a doctor until Tuesday, so, since we just moved here in January and I did not have a local doctor, I called a discreet friend (this is a small town after all) and got a referral.

Tuesday afternoon, I arranged my appointment and met with the doctor where in his exam he felt the (by now) two lumps. He ordered an ultrasound.

Since his clinic is in the local hospital, I had to go through the red tape of paperwork with the hospital to set the ultrasound appointment. About an hour later, one of the techs from Radiology came out and told me that my new doctor, Dr. P, had called and requested that I set an appointment for my ultrasound for 2pm on Wednesday, the next day. (He was working on call in the ER and could not make it. He wanted to be there to perform the ultrasound.)

Wednesday, we had the ultrasound. Important points that I picked up on during the conversation between the radiology tech and the doctor were that there were 2 lumps, and no apparent blood flow to the larger one which they were measuring at approximately 2cm in diameter. My appointment to get the results after the radiologist made his report was on Thursday morning.

The radiologist report recommended that I travel to Odessa for a second opinion. The doctor insisted that I wait while his staff set the appointment in Odessa at MCH Breast Care Center for that Friday.

Not wanting Zoe, who is 10, to sit at home alone all day, she went with me to Odessa on Friday with plans for a lunch date. I bought breakfast for her at Burger King on the way out of town so it felt like a mommy/daughter day out to her. The appointment was set for 11 am.

To keep things light, I had, after the excruciating pain of the mammogram, convinced Zoe to help me play a joke on the technician. After she had prepared the room for the ultrasound and returned to the dressing room to get me for the next step, Zoe looked at her with those big baby blue eyes and asked her, "You are not going to hurt my mommy again are you?" This caused the tech to do some quick stuttering and stammering, but we laughed together about the joke.

When the doctor came into the room to perform the ultrasound, while standing behind the doc, the tech made a comment about feeling like I had 'set her up'. We laughed together, and then, in total seriousness, the doctor looked at me and said, "I get the feeling that you are one of these people who tries to deal with serious situations through the use of humor. However, let me assure you that this technician is a professional. She would never hurt you more than is necessary to perform the needed tests."

To make a long story short, a third lump was found. The three lumps were 3cm, 2cm, and 2cm. (I honestly believe that the TV character of "Bones" was based on this doctor.) She recommended that I have a biopsy A.S.A.P. while telling me again how serious my situation was.

Zoe and I skipped our lunch out, opting to buy some chicken strips for Zoe and a sausage on a stick for me at a convenience store, fill up the tank, and drive the 1.5 hours home. We had just gotten past Monahans when I was connected to my doctor who asked if I could be at the hospital at 3pm for a biopsy. (When they say A.S.A.P. they are not kidding around!)

I dropped Zoe off at the house, made arrangements with a neighbor to check on her, texted Bruce and my son, Zachary, and waited. I can't tell you much of what happened after that other than I have not lost my sense of humor; they were able to remove all 3 tumors; the doctor says they were 'ugly' and looked cancerous; I came home that night; and I will get the pathology results and prognosis on Monday or Tuesday.

I have decided that any woman who voluntarily has breast surgery should have her head examined. . . it is the most painful surgery I have ever had.

Today, Bruce walked with me. I managed to walk 1.7 miles. Not bad for someone who was under-the-knife night before last.

Believe it or not, the thing I am most looking forward to right now . . . the thing that I want more than anything else in the world . . . I want a shower!!! Tonight, I get to remove the support tape, and take that shower. I can hardly wait!

3

IN LAYMAN'S TERMS

Okay Class, to understand cancer, you need to create a few visuals. First, if you have ever run a copier, you know that the older the copier gets, the more likely it is to need maintenance. And if you copy from a copy from a copy, you will experience many variances and deviations from the original. Sometimes, the copier will spit out the occasional blank. Sometimes the copier will jam and crumple your new copies leaving a muddled mess inside. When the cells of your body do this, we call it cancer.

I know you are not going to like hearing this part, but everyone has cancer cells in their body. The only difference between the initial cancer cell and the original copy is that it starts with small variations from the original. Whether the cell continues to mutate and eventually over-reproduce determines whether or not you get CANCER.

The natural world is full of analogies that we can use to demonstrate the difference between the occasional cellular mutation and a full blown cancer. Compare the cells of our bodies with a lush lawn that has a few weeds. You can pull them. You can spray them. You can cut them down. But, they, or others like them are blown in on the wind, floated in as seed in the rain, etc. No matter how well the lawn is cared for, there will be the occasional weed come in. Trees seed in the same way. Seeds blow in or float in, or are carried in and if left unchecked can eventually form a forest. Then, there is the mesquite tree. You can chop it off above the ground, but it sends out deep root runners that, if left unchecked, will start new trees from the roots of the one you thought you got rid of.

Cancer is like that. The doctors have told me that this adenocarcinoma has been in my body for 10-15 years like weeds hiding underneath lush grass. Now, however, it has decided to try and take over the yard, so I began to learn how to fight.

In order to determine how well the cancer is established, today begins a series of medical tests. Within the next two weeks, I will have blood tests, a full cardio workup to determine my ability to handle another surgery, a colonoscopy to check things out on the inside, and a CAT scan of my torso to determine if the cancer has metastasized, or sent out seeds and roots to other organs or the bones of my body. This part is called 'Staging'. From the information obtained in these tests, I will be assigned a Stage number from I-IV with I being best and IV being worst. After all of the tests are run, in 2-3 weeks, I will be scheduled to have a "modified-radical mastectomy". This means that in addition to removing my breast, the doctors will remove approx. 20 lymph nodes and some of the surrounding muscle tissues. (They are researching whether they will build me a new one while they are already there, or have it done at a later date, leaving me lopsided for a while.)

Before he contacted me with the results of the biopsy, the doctor contacted a doctor of oncology (one who specializes in cancer) and they began to draw up the recommended treatment plans. Since I have accepted the recommended oncologist, he is busy going over my pathology reports and will receive copies of all of my new tests so that he can determine and individualize a treatment plan based on my condition (physical and mental) and my stage.

If you have any questions, I will do my best to answer them. For now, though, I am heading for a 7am appointment with a blood lab and cardiologist.

4

LAB TESTS

Part of the process of Staging involves many, many, many tests. In preparation for the surgery, I will go to a cardiologist for a full cardio work up to be sure my heart is strong enough for the surgery. Coming up in the near future, I have a bone scan to check for bone metastases, and a CAT scan to check for tumors in any of my internal organs. Yesterday, I got started with a simple blood test, EKG, and Urinalysis.

Part of going to war against cancer includes dressing for the battle, so I headed to the clinic dressed in my black with pink lettering "Fight like a girl" tee shirt, and baggy hot pink shorts with an elastic waist. I even wore my pink rope cancer ribbon earrings. (Montana Silversmiths. After my husband introduced me to Montana Silversmith's jewelry, Tractor Supply became my favorite jewelry store!)

I was told that I could have the tests run easily if I showed up right at 7 am. It wasn't so much an 'appointment' (the clinic is in the hospital, so the hospital actually does the testing) as it was a suggestion of a time when I would not have as long a wait as I normally have in the afternoons. So, being an early riser, I showed up at 10 till 7 with the idea that I would be quickly in and out.

Since I am accustomed to eating within 30 minutes of getting out of bed, and was unable to eat prior to the blood tests (another reason that 7 am was suggested to me), I grabbed a bottle of Pure Life water from the fridge and drank it to fill in the holes before I left the house. (I probably should have sipped it and carried it with me, but what do I know?) Anyway, I expected to be done and home within an hour or so . . . it's a small town, right . . .

Wrong. As I said earlier, I arrived at 10 minutes before 7. I was prepared with my Kindle, and I sat down to wait. Since I was the ONLY patient there, waiting for the Admissions to open and let the labs know I was there and ready, I looked into the windows of the gift shop and strolled around the lobby to kill time. I am also used to walking in the mornings and just didn't feel like sitting down.

At 7:00, a custodian working in the area took pity on me and asked if he could help me. I explained that I was waiting for admissions. He told me that they were in their office, but hadn't opened their windows yet, and graciously went into the office and informed them that I was there, so I went into the waiting room where the TV was on CNN and the air conditioner was on sub-arctic temperatures to wait for admissions to let "Blood" and "Respiratory" know that I was there and ready.

At 7:15, I decided that a cold room and full bladder were not a good combination, so I again returned to the Lobby to wander and wonder where I could find a public restroom. The custodian again reappeared and being a compassionate fellow, apologized to me for the wait and justified it by saying that he could see the "Blood" lab lady making her hospital rounds. (It was a hit your forehead moment . . . I KNOW that in hospitals blood labs LOVE to wake you up at 7 am and draw blood.) So I sat to read and show myself that I was an understanding person. By 7:30, as I watched the hospital staff shift change; I was beginning to become desperate for a potty.

Finally, at 7:45, the lab tech came in and called my name. I took one look at her and said, "I was beginning to become desperate!"

I followed the diminutive young lady back to the blood lab where she handed me a urine specimen cup and some clean wipe swabs and pointed to the restroom. I smiled and thanked her, reminding her that I was desperate, and headed for the corner door she had pointed out.

As I walked into the small square typical hospital restroom, I noticed several things . . . there was a tree in the back corner behind a leather loveseat both in line with the door, with a sink to the right which was across from the potty in the back right corner. I hollered over my shoulder that I was NOT going to ask what a leather loveseat was doing in a small bathroom. I decided that I didn't want to (although I suspected) know what kind of samples that was used for. I made my way to the potty (finally) in the very small bathroom.

One of the technological wonders/advances that has occurred since my last urinalysis is a nifty, curved, flesh toned, deep cup that screws onto the top of the specimen jar to prevent spillage onto the hand when giving a urine sample. I marveled at that, and then noted that the lab lady had given me a 3-pack of the wipes. Curiously, but mostly needing to pee, I grabbed one from the pack and set to work.

The toilet, as I have said, faced the sink, so facing the sink, I dropped my hot pink shorts and got down to much needed business.

Most people are visual. I am auditory. I have always been auditory, and will always be auditory. I quickly discovered that the major problem with the modern miracle of technology was that I could not HEAR the sound of my pee entering the specimen jar to determine when I was getting close to the top. About the time that realization hit me, the urine began the overflow onto my hand.

I knew that I was not even half finished . . . did I mention that I was DESPERATE . . . and now I was having some SERIOUS overflow issues . . . she should have given me 3-5 jars for this instead of just one! I got myself to stop what I was doing, and poured some of the overflow into the toilet. It was not enough. I poured some more and decided that I needed to find a way to set the cup down NOW without pouring it all over my hot pink shorts which were around my ankles and would need to be passed over to get the overfull specimen cup (which I could not see into because of the miracle of modern technology overflowing from the top) so I decided that the best thing would be to get it to the sink where I could set it down, wash off my dripping hand, and then finish my business.

With pants around ankles, I hobbled to the sink four feet away, sloshing all the way. (By now, I was in a fit of giggles that didn't help hold things steady.) I managed to pull off my plan with only a minimum of sloshing spills (I thought), poured the overflow directly down the drain of the sink, and set the cup with the now seemingly unwieldy miracle of modern technology on the only flat surface...between the hot water knob and the faucet. I unscrewed the miracle of modern technology, threw it into the trash, put the lid on the specimen jar, and washed my hands rapidly all in record time.

Feeling quite proud of my ingenuity and believing that I had maybe only spilled a couple of droplets, I turned to finish my business and discovered that I had left a trail on the floor that resembled what an overeager puppy seeking a favorite visitor might do. I didn't have time to worry about it yet. Grabbing my shorts waistband, I pulled them up to my knees so that they wouldn't drag through the puppy puddle, and rush waddled to finish my business. (Remember, I was DESPERATE!!!)

As I finished my business in a fit of giggles (not wanting to laugh out loud lest the lab tech, who did not have an apparent sense of humor, think she was dealing with a mental patient), it occurred to me. Now I know why the lab tech gives a 3 pack of wipes for a simple urinalysis! They were to clean up the mess made by using the miracle of modern technology!

Sadly, when I pulled up my shorts, they were damp. They must have dragged through my puppy puddles.

I wonder what my next test will be like!

5

MORE TESTS; INTERESTING LESSONS

During the week, when I am travelling to one doctor or another for another round of tests, it feels as if this cancer has always been a part of my life; a part of me. It is not until the weekend when it rears its ugly head with a surreal quality. I guess that is because during the week with the tests and the doctors' offices, I feel like I am actively in the fight. With the down time (which my body really needs and craves by the weekend) there is more time to think and less to act and it becomes just a bit intimidating . . . but that is just perception. It is what it is and I know that my body is continuing the fight. That may be why I am so physically tired by the weekend.

The CAT scan went well. It was an interesting process. I showed up and signed in. After about 30 minutes, a lab tech came and gave me a HUGE jug of barium to drink and told me to drink it and come back in 2 hours. I carried the delightful mixture to the truck and drank it down before driving off. It tasted like it was flavored with coconut . . . without the sweet . . . sort of like skim coconut milk. (This gives a whole new meaning to drinking and driving.) When I got home, I explained to my 10 year old daughter what was going on and we joked about how mommy would glow in the dark that night. (When she became serious and asked if I would really glow in the dark, I told her "only on the inside.")

Upon returning for the CAT scan, I was happy to see one familiar face. It was the same lab tech who had been present when my doctor did the first ultrasound. This gentleman radiates care and concern for the patient, but I worried for him. He is one of those kind souls with the soulful, sorrowful look of a basset hound. When I joke, he just looks at me with his deeply ingrained compassion and it leaves me falling short.

We chatted pleasantly while he inserted the IV (he was very smooth with the needle which I appreciate) and he then went to take the first scans.

For the CAT scan, an IV with iodine is inserted (in conjunction with saline). The iodine reacts with the barium to create a contrast within your cells and allow unique patterns to show, including the outlines of the various internal organs, and the cancer which showed up looking something like spider webs in a haunted house.

After the first round of pictures, I was allowed a small break during which he asked about my biopsy; questions such as who had done it and when. He recognized that this process is travelling much quicker with me than with most because the cancer seems to be so aggressive. If I had had any doubts about the need for the modified radical mastectomy before the CAT, I have none now. To my untrained eye, it looks like the operation should get 85-90 % of the cancer, leaving the rest for chemotherapy. After careful discussion with my husband, we have decided to request that a double mastectomy be done so that we do not have to repeat this process on the other side 4-5 years down the line. (An ounce of prevention; as it was.) I was fortunate to be able to look at my scans even though there was no one who would explain them to me. Technicians are not allowed to share their understanding with the patients. I did feel better after seeing them. To my untrained eye, things are still localized to the tissues of the left side although spidering out rather extensively through the lymph nodes, and we don't need to waste time getting as much of it out as possible.

Our visit to the cardiologist was much more upbeat. The cardio workup, I have been told, is to be sure that my heart is strong enough to withstand the rather major coming surgery. (The cardiologist told me that it would not be quite as bad as my description to him of 'butchering the doe while she lives', but at least he did laugh.) He also assured me that I have hit the lucky jackpot in the doctors who are staffing up my team. He looked in my records and told me that the oncologist that was recommended by my family doctor is one of the best--if not THE BEST in the country in his opinion. He also had very high praise for my doctor who has been with me on this journey and putting me in contact with all of the right people to staff my army.

Stress tests are not what they once were. No treadmills anymore. Now, they thread an IV (3rd one in a week) and insert a contrast agent. About an hour later, they send you through another machine (I am not sure if it is a CAT or MRI) to photo your heart at rest. This is followed by the actual stress test where they inject an agent through the IV which takes your heart to maximum burn. After 1 minute, the staff takes your vitals, and then injects a counter agent which is designed to wipe out the 'racing' drug. (I felt like I had run 5 miles at maximum velocity in just over one minute!) After another 30 minutes, during which they took me for an ultrasound on my heart, they repeat the photo session.

The ultrasound was the most fascinating to both my daughter and me. She was allowed to come and see the pictures of Mommy's heart on the monitor. The tech graciously pointed out to Zoe the four chambers, the valves, blood flow, and explained each thing she was doing. (I think my baby girl thought it was ALMOST as good as watching her comedies on Nick and Disney channels!)

The staff at the oncologist's office is one that I cannot possibly say enough positive things about! They were wonderful. In many ways, it was like a friendly visit to old friends who joke with you and listen and laugh. (With the exception that you would not expect old and dear friends to stab you with needles while joking and listening, and then drugging you and un-drugging you . . . at least not with any of my old crowd!) In short, they made what could have been a frightening experience an enjoyable one.

I have been threaded with IV needles three times in the past week, opened up, stitched back, irradiated internally and photographed in ways I had never before experienced. I still have a bone scan to face on the 20th, but don't expect it to be quite so taxing. Although I did not get to walk yesterday morning due to the drive, I feel like I got in a 5 mile run, and I slept better last night than I have since first discovering the lumps in my breast 13 days ago. Although today is only the 16th, I have spent some portion of 11 days of this month with medical professionals in one capacity or another. I feel blessed. I have the support of a wonderful army to help me fight this fight, and you, my friends and family standing on the sidelines cheering me on and waiting to pick me up if I should fall. Thank you. You are wonderful!

6
ADDRESSING THE ISSUE

I had a decent weekend, although it was a bit hard. Bruce had to work on Saturday. When he came back home, one of the guys he works with had graciously gifted him with a cold. He had a sore throat, muscle aches, was feverish, and would not come within 5 feet of me.

It was the first time in our 22 years together that I could not comfort and take care of him. There is too great a risk that a cold now would leave me unable to have the surgery within the next week or so. So, I had to satisfy myself with going to Wal-Mart and buying massive quantities of vitamin C, Echinacea, and anything else I could think of that might make him heal and feel better more quickly. (I am kind of hooked on his kisses and not being able to have any this weekend . . . or to snuggle up close at night . . . was very hard.) He was right though...right now, the risk is too great to be messed with. He did insist that I grab up a lot of vitamin C for me too, so that I can work at fighting off any potential problems before they arise. He reasoned that since we know that the cancer is in my lymphatic system, an ounce of prevention could be a real life-saver.

All of that aside, I had been planning to inform my boss of my condition when I had more information to hand him . . . like a date for the surgery, and possibly information about the stage and what my specific cancer is. My timetable was bumped up though, through intervention of a certain 10 year old girl.

Saturday, while Bruce was at work, my daughter and I went to the grocery store to stock up on 'healthy food'. We looked at, discussed, and bought beautiful veggies in the fresh food section, chicken and fish in the fresh meats, Ensure for Mommy and Daddy, fruit juices for her, and of course the necessities such as toilet paper and paper plates (or as we like to call them around here--fine china.) We had gone the full circuit when my daughter decided that she wanted to have ham sandwiches for her lunches this week. Since we did not have any sandwich meat, we headed back to the Deli meat section of the store.

I was very happy to see the beautiful lady who is my boss's secretary. She is the type of lady who radiates. I called to her and she turned. With a smile, she called out, "Jamie Batson! How are you?"

Before I could say a word, my ten year old, well-meaning daughter, piped up from behind me, "She has cancer!"

There followed an exchange of information that I was not quite ready for, but was able to relate. I then found that the best time to come and visit with my boss about the situation would be around 7am on Monday morning. She told me that he has been out of town visiting family, and I explained to her that I did not want to call and tell him about it over the phone . . . that I felt it would be better to pass along in person. I told her that I would be there first thing on Monday morning, and again apologized to her for finding out about this situation the way that she did.

In discussing with my daughter what she did, I did tell her that she reminds me much of myself at her age. I too tended to blurt things that I knew, rather than allowing the adults to have the adult conversation without added information being thrown out there for them. (How do you get angry at your child for being too much like yourself?) I think that she understands, but the timetables have now been moved up on telling people, so it is about to be thrown out there for the world to know, and deal with.

I wish that all of my experiences could be like the one I wrote about in "Lab Test"...with the exception of the damp shorts . . . but I already know that cancer is a word that strikes fear into the hearts and minds of most people, and it carries with it a wide emotional range. Life right now is a bit like being on a rollercoaster in the dark. You don't know when the next turn is coming . . . whether it will take you up, down, or spin you around, but you know that it is coming.

7

MR. TOAD'S WILD RIDE

I am reminded of the children's story of "Mr. Toad's Wild Ride" which is a parody of the ups and downs of life. It feels some days like I am on that untamed and untamable ride. It is moving too fast to jump off, so I just need to keep hanging on.

Yesterday morning, I walked to the high school to get my walking in, and to do the unenviable task of telling my Principal and Assistant Principal of my condition. I made the walk in 10 minutes, so I was there just before 7am and managed to beat them there, although the beautiful secretary I told you about yesterday was already getting started on her day. She and I chatted for a couple of minutes, and then I went to my classroom to look at what I needed to get done before the surgery in order to have my classroom in shape. After moving a couple of things around, I headed back to the office.

When I came into the office, Mr. A and Mr. S were setting up the US and Texas flags in the office for the week. We said good morning, and I told them that I had something to tell them and since there was no easy way to do it, they should just keep working on their tasks while I talked. While they worked, I explained the situation, including what little I do know about my condition and how very much I don't know. The two men were mostly silent and Mrs. B asked questions that she felt might help the two men to understand. Mr. S even asked a couple of questions. I could see that Mr. A was greatly disturbed by my news. He went into his office and faced his computer with his back to the door for a few minutes while Mrs. B and I continued to discuss the cancer, and what I still needed to do for the staging, and the FMLA paperwork that will need to be completed at some point in the near future.

I have noticed that while women are quick to discuss and ask questions, men tend to be at a loss for words. This is okay. Abraham Lincoln said, "It is better to be silent and be thought a fool than to speak and remove all doubt." My heart goes out to them though . . . especially when they are usually quick witted with their comments and input as I know Mr. A to be.

From his desk, Mr. A finally turned and faced me. He, in all earnestness, looked me in the eye and told me that he really hates that I am going through all of this. He went on and told me that he has a niece who is about to have reconstruction surgery from a similar situation. I told him to have her look at the saltwater implants since I have read and heard many wonderful things about them for the reconstruction. He promised to pass on the information.

Mrs. B and I resumed talking about the paperwork and substitutes for when I am unable to be at work . . . possibly finding one person who would be willing to be my right hand as needed to help keep the classroom as stable as possible. After a few more minutes, Mr. A came out of his office.

In answer to what I need from them, I told them to please not lose the sense of humor and camaraderie that we have always shared. As Mr. A (who is quite bald) came back into the main office, I looked at him and grinned and said, "Hey. I have an idea. Why don't you and I go bald together this year?"

It had the desired effect, and he was once again smiling when I left the office.

As those of you who have decided to join me on this wild ride know, I had good news yesterday afternoon. When I took my FMLA paperwork to the clinic and found out that my CAT results were in. The prognosis is very good. Results showed that the cancer is localized to the left breast and lymph nodes on that side. In discussing with my doctor these results, we also had an opportunity to discuss information exchanged between him and the oncologist. While we are not sure until after the staging and surgeries are complete what the next step will be, he told me that because of the aggressive nature demonstrated by this cancer that I will probably have radiation, and possibly have chemotherapy. The deciding variable is whether the pathology shows that my cancer is sensitive to one or more hormones . . . meaning estrogen, progesterone, or HER2. With the way that it is behaving, the doctors feel that it will be reactive to one or more of these even though I have not had the hormone making equipment since 2005. If it has fooled them and does not respond to any of the three, which would make it triple negative, and much harder to treat. (He did stress that with my medical history they expect it to be an estrogen responsive cancer.) We also had the opportunity to set up my initial consultation with the surgeon for July 28.

This morning was wonderful. I headed out for my walk with the intention of making a full mile on the track . . . or 4 laps. As I was walking my third lap, I was just thinking how wonderful it would be to be like Forrest Gump . . . just waking and walking with my friends and family until this cancer was beaten. As I came around the back half of my fourth lap, a lady I had never met came rushing across the street to the track shouting to me, asking if I was going to continue walking. I told her that I was on my last lap, but if she wanted to walk with me that I thought I had another lap in me. She came onto the track and introduced herself to me as 'Rose'.

Rose told me that she suffers from depression and that she wanted to walk, but that she hates to walk alone. I pointed to the many birds and dragonflies around us and told her that I never feel alone when I am walking . . . that I can always sense that none of us is really walking alone, but that I was more than happy to have her walk with me. We easily walked and talked like two old friends becoming reacquainted after a long time apart. I told her my story and she told me hers. It was as easy to visit and get to know one another as breathing. We agreed to meet in the morning at 7 am to walk together again.

We parted ways and as I was walking home, I received a call from the cardiologist's office. It was more good news. My heart is strong and ready and able to handle the surgery. After a brief discussion of which doctor is doing what (I am beginning to need a program to keep up with them all) we ended our conversation. Before hanging up, I asked the young lady to give Dr. G1 a message for me. I asked her to tell him that the stress test made me feel like I had gone from 0-60 in 5.2. She laughed and promised to pass on the message. She also told me that he had said for me to just keep doing what I am doing and I will be fine.

My outlook is good. I am seeing positive messages everywhere I look. As I sit here typing and sucking on Vitamin C drops, I looked down at the wrapper. Typed in the center of the wrapper are the words "Conquer Today". I believe I will. I walked 3.17 miles this morning. Today is a great day to be alive!

8
OUTSIDE OF THE BOX

There are many parallels between education and medically treating the outside quotient . . . the unknown factor, the cancer of the body, and the student who does not quite fit in. In our quest for human understanding, we tend to use statistics to try and determine patterns that we can use to neatly fit everyone in every circumstance into. With our predetermined interpretation of problems based on the 'average' person and their responses to stressful situations, we struggle to fit each person and situation neatly into a preordained pattern of behavior and response. However, not everyone fits neatly into the box, and some of us resist it with kicking and screaming . . . or laughter.

Being just as guilty of looking for those patterns, we tend to seek them and see them in everyday life. For example, my father grew up as the middle son of all boys. I am the middle daughter of all girls. Thus, I can see and establish the pattern that satisfies my need to draw some parallels. Another trait that I share with my father is a certain 'irreverence' toward situations that most people find to be times to join in the ancient art of wailing and gnashing of teeth.

For example, many years ago, when I was living in El Paso, my father's favorite aunt passed- away. He came to her funeral which was a graveside service. Standing in the overcast weather with the smoldering grey skies above us, surrounded by the last dozen of her grey haired surviving friends, we chose to stand together at the edge of the artificial turf carpet that had been rolled out under a canopy for the memorial service and the traditional lowering of the casket into the ground. To the tune of these dozen ancient friends stifled tears, my dad leaned over to me and quietly whispered, "I wonder who we are standing on."

With stifled giggles, I responded, "I don't know, but I hope that they had a strong coffin," and pointed to the marker where the only thing that could be clearly seen was the date of death in 1836.

Another example is when in a discussion on Skype with my parents when I was telling them about my initial exam, I made the mistake of saying something about when the doctor" got his hands on it", meaning the lump, but since I was talking about a breast exam, it made my dad demonstrate his use of this irreverent humor we share.

My husband has learned through the years to share openly this irreverent humor as well. Last September when I had my gallbladder removed unexpectedly, he held my hand tenderly and said, "Jamie, you have got to stop trying to lose weight by having your internal organs removed one at a time."

I have had similar moments through the years, and many opportunities to handle situations with this same outside of the box attitude that has served me well so far in life. Evidently, I must be projecting it now in my attitude about the cancer.

I went yesterday to have my bone scan to check for any metastasizes into the bones of my body. (Areas where the cancer may have spread) We are continuing to hope that since the cancer has not spread to my internal organs, it will not have spread into my bones. (Our reasoning is simple . . . bones are harder to penetrate, so it should feed on something softer first, right?--We realize that this is partially hopeful thinking, but we plan to keep thinking this way until something proves us wrong.)

The bone scan was the most pleasant of all of my tests for staging. My scheduled time was noon, so we arrived, and met with the technician. She was another lovely lady who proved to be quite the warrior against cancer. She injected me with the 'contrast' (great . . . more radioactive waste for my body to dispose of . . .) and sent us to lunch.

I have been tracking my exercise and caloric intake on livestrong.com, and had arrived at the Neurosciences Clinic with a deficit. Rose and I had such a wonderful time walking and talking that I did not keep up with my laps and ended up walking 4.66 miles before breakfast . . . burning off enough calories that I was starting the day with a 500 calorie deficit when we headed out. Anyway, I had promised Zoe a lunch date at Jason's Deli.

One of the things that the technician insisted on was that I drink more fluids than I thought I could hold in order to help the fresh batch of radioactive contrast agent to do its job. So, in addition to my tomato basil soup (love that stuff) and salad bar, I drank at least 32 oz. of iced tea. Zoe ordered a cup of the tomato basil soup, which she ate, a Frito pie special, of which she ate half, and five ice cream cones, which she insisted were healthy because they tasted more like frozen yogurt.

Thankful that I was NOT wearing my hot pink shorts after drinking all of that tea, we headed back to the Neurosciences Clinic for our 2:30 return time.

I had been told to go to the restroom before coming back into the office for the scan so that we would not need to stop in the middle of the scan to go to the restroom. "I am a good girl" (that quote is for you, Mother) and try to do as I am told when it comes to medical activities. Not surprisingly, the first question that the technician, we will call her Caroline, asked me was whether or not I had gone to the bathroom.

Before we began the test, which consists of lying very still (sleeping is allowed) on a very slow- moving table while your body is scanned, Caroline asked me many questions from a questionnaire, and a few of her own. It was only upon reflection that I realized her puzzled looks were because I apparently am treating my diagnosis with outside of the box thinking.

After asking if I had ever had a bone scan before, she looked at my calm, yet curious face and stated, "You have had a great many women in your family go through this, haven't you."

When I answered her by telling her that I am the one and only, it was her turn to look shocked and curious. She then followed up with, "You have had many incidences of fibrocystic disease then." (Fibrocystic disease is a hereditary condition in which women develop lumps in their breasts. They are non-cancerous when associated with the disease.)

To which I told her that I am the only woman in my family who has not had fibrocystic disease. She really looked confused then!

As the tests were being run, she seemed to enjoy showing and telling my daughter, "See! Your Mama sure is a boney woman, isn't she?" (I suppose that somewhere deep down inside that is true, but I have not looked 'boney' from the outside for a long, long time!)

The actual tests took about 45 minutes during which I managed a couple of cat naps. She also took a screen that had been fastened above the moving table and positioned it so that I could see the scans too....when they were not scanning my skull.

Carolyn was just as stubborn about not telling what she knows as all of the other techs. (To them it is called "professionalism" . . . to my impatience to know . . . "frustration".) But she was equally polite. She was continuing to give me puzzled looks as we left.

I had to sleep on it to realize that, like the kid in the classroom that most of the teachers have no clue how to work with, I address my cancer with an outside of the box thinking. Since nothing about this experience has been in accordance with what the textbook teaches (i.e., it started out painful, widespread but not metastasized, no family history, no correlating conditions, I am not scared to death but accepting to the point of irreverent) many of these medical professionals find me to be something of an enigma.

I definitely do not fit the mold, and I am very happy that way. I refuse to let this cancer define who I am. I prefer to redefine the cancer. After all, it is what it is, and I am what I am, and we do not have to be one and the same. I plan to laugh this insidious enemy into oblivion and just keep on keeping on!

9

MARKING TIME

Wow! What a wonderful weekend we had meeting up with classmates from 30 years ago! It was interesting to see how many people grew up to become their parents! (In looks only, of course.)

In regards to the cancer, this weekend I learned that I will never willingly put on a bra again. Sports bras, and built in bras are alright, but I have about decided that there is a correlation between underwire and breast cancer. After just a few hours of wearing one to the events, I would go back to the house and find that the knots in my breast had knotted themselves again around where the 'support' of the bra sat, and the pain would be back. Another interesting and somewhat disturbing phenomenon was that the top and center of my chest would feel somewhat numb . . . sort of like when you sit on your foot and cut of the circulation to the point that it 'falls asleep'. The numbness is on a list of things to discuss with the Surgeon on Thursday when I go in. It is fairly constant, but was much more pronounced for about 12 hours after wearing the bra on Friday and Saturday nights.

I should know the date for the surgery on Thursday afternoon. We are ready to get it done and get to the position that we feel like we are actively at war with this stuff. Even though I read and research and am aware of all the negative possibilities, all I can see and think of are all of the positives. It has been this way with all of the surgeries that I have needed through the years to prolong my life. I already know that in pre-op, I do not behave like the 'average' surgical patient. My attitude about it is one of looking forward to the change in the pain from an unhealthy pain/discomfort to one that is healthy. There is a difference in the two types of pain. I don't know if everyone can feel the difference in the two types (healthy vs. unhealthy), or if this is something somewhat unique to me.

There are two research studies that I would like to be able to find online. One deals with the correlation of underwire to breast cancer, and the other deals with the number of people who are able to actively distinguish between healthy and unhealthy pain.

When I talk about healthy pain, I am referring to the pain that is there after the sick parts are removed...it is the pain that comes with healing; with regaining health after having the unhealthy removed. Things falling into the unhealthy category would be things like a ripe appendix, a gallbladder attack, and the ovarian cysts that I once did battle with, the torn meniscus. The healthy pain is the recovery after the surgery; after the appendix, gallbladder, cysts, or meniscus are removed and the pain is just the pain associated with healthy healing. To me, the 'healthy pain' of post-surgery is like the feeling that surges through my legs after my morning power walk; the tingling feel of the blood flowing unfettered through veins and arteries sending oxygen to muscle and bone. That is the feeling that I am looking forward to feeling. I will welcome with joy the feelings and sensations that will come along with whatever additional treatments after the surgery come along because I know that these are the sensations that will indicate to me that my body is working hard to fix the problems that come from the cancer.

To help prepare my body for recovery, I continue to walk in the mornings. Rose and I walked this morning 2.81 miles. It was reviving after the long drive to and from the reunion and temporary changes in routine that came with the trip. The reunion gave me many happy memories that I will pour through in my mind over the weeks and months to come, and help me with the mental healing process just as continuing to walk with Rose will do for my body.

10
DOING THE RESEARCH

After stating that I would like to find some studies about the correlation between underwire bras and cancer, and healthy pain vs. unhealthy pain yesterday, I set out to do the research. What I found was rather interesting.

On the issue of healthy pain vs. unhealthy pain, there is some information, but primarily associated with sports and exercise sites. The primary examples were the differences between normal muscle aches developed through a buildup in the muscle of lactic acid vs. the pain of tears and strains. There was nothing that I could find about the pain of the before and after surgery that I mentioned in my last post.

However, I found quite a bit in the area of correlating wearing of underwire bras with cancer. In 1995, a book called "Dressed to Kill" was published that draws some rather convincing conclusions about a correlation between the restrictions of wearing bras...especially with underwire...and breast cancer.

When researching this online, I have found a split in the numbers of organizations that agree with the possibilities presented in the book. The standard party line presented by all of the cancer agencies is that the correlation is a myth because the study was not conducted by professional cancer researchers. They will follow their party line with a statement that there have been no 'scientific studies' done that would show or dispute a correlation between the two.

In repeatedly reading this party line, I am reminded of the late 1800's where it was common practice to place babies in tightly laced corsets at birth because they were born with weak back muscles. This practice was encouraged by the medical community and lead to much larger health issues down the line. The practice was not suspended until a medical person finally stepped up and did a study that showed the long term problems faced by adults who had been laced up since infancy. (Sometimes I find the 'scientific snobbery' regarding common sense really aggravating!) Since there are no plans among the scientific community to conduct a study on the possible correlation, each of us must come to our own conclusions based on what little is available.

I did my walking this morning with just me and God. Rose was under the weather and didn't feel like making the trip. I walked 2.86 miles, enjoying the light breeze and cooler morning temperatures. Keeping busy while waiting for test results keeps me from thinking about the cancer too much, but the time that I spend between doctors while waiting on those results also allows me to go and take care of some business. Zoe and I went to her new school today and met with her principal and counselors to set up her support network, so it has been a busy day. Tomorrow, we will go to the school and set up my classroom so that it will be easier to start the year . . . with the understanding that lifting and moving things will probably be disallowed for a while. For now, I'll go make tuna salad for supper and feed my family. Everything is going to work out alright.

11

Countdown to a Cure

It has a name. Many things about the name are as positive as can be. Some of the information is not what we had hoped, but we will make the best of it because it is what it is. The name of the cancer I have is "Infiltrating Ductal Carcinoma."

Of the three lesions removed at my lumpectomy, one was infiltrating ductal carcinoma. Two were Ductal Carcinoma in Situ. From all that I have read, the two that were DCIS are considered to be stage 0. In other words, once they were removed, it was over for them. The battle that we are waging is with the Infiltrating Ductal Carcinoma. It is the one that has spread to my lymph glands, and, yes, probably to my sternum.

It took quite a bit of work to get the surgeon to admit that last bit. When I asked him directly about the results of the bone scans, he hedged like a lifelong politician. He kept telling me that the bone scans that count are the ones that are done in 6 months after the chemo and radiation have had a chance to work their magic. I choose to follow his positive line of thought until proven otherwise. He also refuses to remove the right breast until and unless the oncologist has made a recommendation to do it.

Several times in our discussion, he had to pause and think about his answers because I would say or do things that would catch his sense of humor. (It is nice to have a surgeon who can recognize and appreciate irony as a humor tool!) His positive plan is to remove what is cancerous, but leave what can be cosmetically nice after a rebuild is done. He was very positive about us catching this at a beatable stage. He told me that of all the cancer's I could have come up with, so far we are very lucky. When I asked about the hormone receptors and how I rated on those, he did not yet have those results, so he called his nurse back into the room and instructed her to contact the lab in Dallas (didn't know parts of me had been sent that far afield) and get the reports stat so that I could be informed enough to continue my internet research. He seems to understand that I want to battle this in an informed manner. I greatly appreciate his professional manner.

In preparation for this visit, I wrote out a list of questions that I wanted answers to. The only one that he hesitated and tried to bluff his way around was the one about the results of the bone scan. After I asked him very directly about my sternum, he directly gave me the answers that I was seeking. He went on to say that an initial bone scan can often show false positives due to reflections of the agent in concentrated areas of the cancer. He explained in detail what the surgery on Monday would entail, listing (for those of you in the business) that he would be doing a "level II mastectomy" and that the number of lymph nodes that required removal was the most important last step in the staging process. (My boss insisted that I also ask how many times the doctor has performed this surgery. The answer was over 100 times during his residency in Chicago, followed by another hundred in the lead in Chicago. He estimated 50-75 more since he relocated to Texas.)

Interestingly, when I later met with the surgical assistant for my 'pre-op pep talk', I mentioned that Zoe and I had gone online to Google Images yesterday to look at Mastectomies so that she would be better prepared for what was about to happen to her mommy. While searching under mastectomy, we found an actual photo of breast cancer. It looked like rancid cottage cheese. When I mentioned this to the young man in the surgery department, he stated that quite often, in fact most of the time, cancer resembles foods. Knowing that we are what we consume, I am seriously thinking that I may remove cottage cheese from my diet! (The thought of it fermenting in my body after seeing that photo is a great diet incentive!)

My next worry is how unbalanced I am about to be. (Physically, I mean...the mental side of imbalance has always been there and I know how to live with that!) Talk about lopsided . . . one side of me will remain a DDD, and the other will be rather flat in comparison. I have been looking at prostheses, and have yet to find one that clocks in quite that large. (God does have a sense of humor!) The doctor also told me that he plans to work very carefully on leaving a minimal scar so that the plastic surgeon in 6-8 months will have a 'clean palate' to work with in making Bruce's toys 'pretty' again!

The surgery is scheduled for Monday, August 1 at noon. (When the gentleman in surgery called to verify the time, the nurse told him that it is not at noon . . . it is at 12:00pm.) It is what it is, and now it is time to research, learn, and 'fight like a girl'!

12
My Foibles

As I sit here mentally preparing myself for another surgery, I am thinking about how we are all neurotic to various degrees. It seems to be part of the human condition.

I remember years ago sitting in a teacher's lounge and listening to teachers discussing the quirks of their mothers. One of the teachers told us that when she was growing up, her mother required them to carefully and neatly fold all of their dirty clothes before placing them into the laundry basket. The folded clothes were later sorted into neatly folded piles by color and material prior to washing, and then placed into the washing machine still folded. It sounded so ridiculous to us, and we were all laughing in disbelief.

It brought to mind times in my childhood when we would work feverishly in the evening to vacuum and dust, and clean our rooms because the maid was coming the next day to clean. Mother explained to us that she did not want the maid to think that we were messy people. Another thing that I love about my mother was the way that she would wash and style her hair in preparation for her appointment to have her hair washed, cut and styled at the hairdresser.

These funny little quirks are endearing qualities that individualize us and bring smiles to our faces when we think back in time. In short, other's neurosis can make us laugh out loud, but we tend to overlook and try to disguise our own; believing that others don't see them for what they really are...the unique quirks of our minds that those that love us find both frustrating and endearing.

Early in our marriage, Bruce trained me to never expect to receive flowers unless he had done something that I would think was very, very bad. One day, he showed up with a handful of beautiful carnations. The first words out of my mouth were, "What did you do?"

It turned out that in his job at the time as a lineman working on high energy electrical distribution lines, they had been working behind a florist shop when the florists were throwing out the old flowers. He and the other men on his crew went 'dumpster diving' and brought the women in their lives lovely batches of flowers. I thought it was a sweet gesture, and enjoyed the flowers immensely, especially since they were not to make up for some unimaginable offense.

Mixed in with my thoughts of others sits an awareness of my own foibles. I find myself feeling rather sad that I will never be able to donate blood again. Also, over the years, Bruce and I had discussed how we wanted to have this shell we each live in treated after we are no longer inhabiting it. My plan was always to donate my organs to those who needed them to keep on living and improve their quality of life. That was before my systems decided to rebel and I ended up having so many surgeries: an ovary and tube, appendix, hysterectomy with the last ovary and tube, gallbladder, and now a breast. I am coming to grips with the fact that due to my diagnosis, I am donating those organs to science while still using the body that housed them. Hopefully, these experiences will teach the doctors and scientists things that they can use to help other people later, on down the line. It is just as well that this has happened...I mean the cancer...because I was rapidly running out of organs that could have been useful to others later on, and I plan to spend many more years using up those organs that I have left. (I don't think that there are many calls for 90-100 year old hearts, lungs, eyes, etc . . .)

If it sounds like I am down, or depressed, please don't believe that is where I am. In truth, I am somewhat panicked. My folks are coming to our house to help out as I am having the surgery and recovering. With them coming to help out, I find myself, in a parody of my mother's desire to clean before the maid comes, trying to work very hard to have little for them to help out with while they are here. I need to stop typing and go sweep and mop. After all, the apple does not fall far from the tree.

13
Descent of the Vultures

It is a sad fact of life that every family has them. Some families have few. Others have many. Some families are even composed entirely of them. Sadly, they show themselves early and hard when you announce that you have cancer. I am talking about vultures.

Vultures are carrion birds that feed on the recently dead. In the animal kingdom, they wait, circling above, for the death to occur. Human vultures begin to circle just as quickly . . . marking the things that they want that belong to the person whom they are watching; waiting for them to die. From the perspective of the person with cancer, this is perhaps one of the most disconcerting events that occurs in the progression of the disease.

For the sake of anonymity, I will not disclose the real names of my vultures, nor their relationship to me. I have hesitated to make this part of my story because I find it so distasteful that people to whom I am related would behave this way, but it is a very real part of dealing with a severe illness.

The day before my mastectomy, my parents came down to help out with my daughter while I had my surgery and recovery time. Unannounced, and unexpected, another relative showed up with them. For the sake of privacy, we will call her Essie. I will not tell you her real name or her relationship to me. Maybe by now she has figured out that she should be embarrassed by her behaviors that day. Just one day prior to my major surgery. (Last time we talked about it, she was still trying to blame her behavior on me.)

In addition to showing up unexpectedly to our little home, Essie brought with her a dog. He was a delightful little dog, but our landlord (we rent) had a very strict "no pets" policy. (Goldfish were not even to be allowed in the home!) We had done our best to treat our landlord well in hopes that he would be kind to us in turn. When we expressed concern about having a dog in the house, she responded that our landlord would just need to "get over it".

Things did not start out too badly. Essie was bouncing off of the walls jubilantly. About an hour into the visit, I was summoned to have a private conversation with her in the garage. The conversation went something like this.

"I have everything figured out," Essie began, "I will move in here with you, raise your daughter, Zoe, and take care of your husband, Bruce. I will even be the substitute in your classroom. That way, when your students act up, I will tell them to straighten up because I even live with you and you will know what they are up to!"

Clearing my throat and choosing my words carefully, I replied, "I appreciate the offer, but that is not what I need right now."

Essie quipped, "Why not?"

"Because, we would end up killing each other."

"Get over it! That was in high school. We have both grown up since then."

(Things were starting to get tricky for me in how I answered.) "Not entirely . . . if we are being honest with each other," I replied.

"Give me one example," demanded Essie.

"A couple of weeks ago, "I responded, "There was a social game on Facebook where you copied and pasted the request for your friends to list their favorite memory of the person making the post. I posted it, and you typed in that your fondest memory of me was the time you physically assaulted me. I removed the entire post as soon as I saw your response. It concerns me that your fondest memory is of an assault on me and that now you want me to invite you into my home. I did not remove the post because it made me look bad. It made YOU look really bad, and I removed it out of concern for you."

(And now here I am still trying to protect her from herself! I can be rather silly sometimes.)

That was when the screaming and cussing started. I realize that Essie has a diagnosed mental condition, but that should not excuse the behavior that followed. She proceeded to prove me right about the killing each other part.

The yelling began . . . and the cussing. My daughter, who was just ten years old at the time, was in tears. She had never heard anyone scream at her mother that way . . . and use language that would make many a sailor blush!

The tirade escalated until finally she screamed at me, "You are making this all about you."

You could have heard a pin drop in the house as I, in puzzlement at the logic being shown, responded, "This time it IS all about me."

Essie then did the unforgivable. Standing between my daughter and myself, she screamed at me, "You stupid, furling birch!" (Only, she used the actual curse words.) "I hope you DIE on the operating table tomorrow."

Never before, nor since, in my lifetime have I thrown someone out of my home. I did then though. What kind of a person screams things like that at a mother in front of her young daughter who, up until that moment, had probably not realized that the surgery to fix things might also kill? (The answer is that it is the vultures . . . the people who are circling; waiting to see what they can get from your illness . . . and setting themselves to be first in line at your death.)

Following my surgery the next day, as they brought me out of the recovery room and were taking me to my new home away from home for the next few days, my family had the nurse stop the gurney so that they could tell me that Essie was really sorry about her previous behavior and could she come to the room to see how I was doing.

I responded, "What do I care . . . I am on morphine!"

Many months later, at the next family gathering, Essie came to me, very drunk, and apologized. She said, "I am sorry that we had that disagreement. You just didn't understand what I was offering."

14
Surgery

The prelude to the surgery included the prerequisite family drama . . . seems like anything worthwhile must have a bit of that . . . but it has been addressed in another chapter. We can call it life's lessons learned. Let's just suffice it by saying it happened, and we all got past it successfully.

We headed to the hospital early. There was some confusion since the surgeon had told me to be there at 10am, and the surgical team had told me to be there at 11am for my noon surgery. We decided to hedge our bets and get there early in hopes of having the 'festivities' start on time. True to the word of the surgical team, we were escorted back to the surgical prep room shortly before 11am.

In the prep room, I was given a well-ventilated, fashionable gown to wear, and while I answered questions and was poked and prodded like a pin cushion, Mother and Daddy slept in their rolly chairs while Zoe zoomed about in hers like a ride at Six-Flags, and Bruce listened in to questions and answers about the pending surgery. It was a repeat performance for most of the members of my surgical team since most were present for the rush lumpectomy/biopsy that had been done on July 8th. Luckily, they already had experienced (and knew to expect) my 'quick-wit' and sometimes biting humor about the situation.

I can honestly say that I really remember nothing from the operating room after transferring to the operating table, and having a 'minty-fresh' gas mask placed on my face. My next memories were in the recovery room. It seems that I always come to in mid-sentence with the person watching over me there, and I always have a moment of panic. We always seem to have been involved in an in-depth conversation, and I have NO CLUE what it is we are discussing . . . a very disorienting feeling. Shortly after that "Oh, Lord, what are we talking about" moment, my doctor, Dr. P, came into the room and told me that he had met with my family already and told them what he was about to tell me, but that I would not remember our conversation and my family could fill me in. (Being me, I took that statement as a challenge and recited the conversation back to him when he visited me in my room the next day, word for word.)

Dr. P told me that they had gotten all of the cancer. He then repeated ALL of the cancer. HOWEVER (don't you just love it when that 'however' shows up in medical information?), there were several 'hard' spots in the muscle wall of my chest that they were afraid might be new positions that the cancer was trying to develop. They took biopsies of these to have pathology check and see. He also said that they dug and dug and dug through my lymph nodes. While the CAT scan showed the lymph nodes to be fairly eaten up by the cancer, they only found ONE that appeared to be infected. (We are still celebrating that news!)

Shortly after the visit with Dr. P, I was released to my stay in room 25 for the duration of this trip.

The rooms in our local hospital are large and well situated . . . other than the poor planning of placing the hospital bed where it faces the mirror over the sink so that the first horror the patient sees upon waking is his/her own pale-skinned, pain-filled face. (I suppose that is to scare you into having higher blood pressure when they come in to check vitals.) Visitors do have plenty of room to visit. Room 25 was approximately the size of my living room at home. Thankfully, there was not a loveseat in the bathroom.

There were two issues that were the most difficult about coming back from the surgery. The first was the issue of that first trip to the bathroom. The second was (and still is) the issue of the drainage bags.

Having had an IV placing fluids into my body since about 11am, I was well hydrated. The anesthesia had left me with a dry mouth, however, and Zoe was busily shoving ice chunks into my mouth in an effort to ease my dry throat. Add to that the liquid dinner I was given at 5:30 (best chicken broth I can remember ever having . . . it certainly was not as good the next morning at breakfast) and the two sodas that I requested and received, and I was ready for my first trip to the bathroom by about 7:30 that night.

After so many surgeries, I guess that I decided that I was an old hand at the process. When it was time, I was under instructions from the hospital staff that I was to call for a nurse when I needed to go that first time. Knowing that a nurse would be there was not as much of a comfort though as knowing that Bruce would still be there for me. He was, and would be, by my side as I made that first trip which signals an important step in post-surgical recovery.

Many years ago, in 1991 as a matter of fact, I had come off of a horse named Doobie. The latigos had snapped on the saddle while Doobie was in a hard run and when he turned, there was nothing to keep me on his back. My injuries had been extensive enough that I had severely injured my hip, and shoulder, and knew that I had a concussion when I saw about 15 trucks sitting in front of 15 houses when Bruce tried to help me get up and back inside. It took him about 1 ½ hours to get me the 200 feet from where I landed into the house because I kept taking two steps and passing out. This trip would revive those memories for us both.

The first trip to the bathroom after a mastectomy is a process. It takes quite a bit of time under the best circumstances, but is a matter of working through the pain. Planning ahead to meet the timelines is very important. The first step in this process is requesting pain medication and a nurse to witness your achievement. (Mommy...I went potty by myself! I'm a big girl now!) The nurse will also disconnect the many machines and fluids that are keeping you tethered to the bed. It also helps to have the big, strong man you love there to catch you if you should need someone to catch you. (This part is rather hard on the big, strong man, though, and you may feel bad about any new grey in his hair after the fact!)

The second step involves sitting up unsupported in the hospital bed. If you become dizzy, this step will need to be repeated...in fact if you become dizzy, all steps will need to be repeated from this one on. If, however, you are successful in sitting unsupported for 3-5 minutes, you can move on to the next step which involves turning your body to where your feet hang off of the bed and sitting unsupported with feet dangling for what is beginning to feel like an eternity (because you really need to go pee by now!)

After passing the dangling feet test, you are allowed to move forward and place feet firmly on the floor while remaining seated, unsupported but for the hands of your loved ones on your arms and fearing that they will hurt you, tending to be too gentle to offer much physical support. That is alright though since the pain has now awakened and is sitting up with you to say, "Hello."

Now, things begin to speed up. It is finally time to stand and walk the 2000-3000 steps it takes to get across the 10 feet of open floor to the bathroom door. As I stood, and Bruce lovingly leaned in to support me, I whispered in his ear, "This may be like the Doobie incident. Pay attention and I promise to let you know as quickly as I can."

Through the pain, I am laughing at myself. I am tottering to another hospital restroom with an elephant sized need to pee while wearing a truly backless gown, and I have on my hot pink underwear. I may hurt, but the irony was almost enough to elicit a giggle!

After depositing approximately 5 gallons of fluid (I told you that I really needed to go), it was later determined that my full bladder was all that was keeping my blood pressure up to a decent level. I was able to stand while Bruce and the nurse pulled up my hot pink undies, and took about 2 steps when I told Bruce, "Now!!! It's NOW!!!" and I felt his arms go around me.

I know that they were able to reseat me on the potty rather than spill me on the floor because I came to on the potty. I have been told that I was out for approximately 30 minutes and that more nurses and a chair had been summoned. The nurses arrived shortly afterwards with the chair. We (when I say we, I mean the nurses and Bruce) were able to move me to the chair, and then transfer me from the chair to the bed with no further incidents.

In straightening out the 'why' of it taking so long, we discovered (after-the-fact) that while the nurse who was in the restroom with me would press the call button (there in the restroom) to summon help, and help would arrive; unaware of the drama playing out on the potty, my mother and Zoe, who were sitting beside the door to the hall would tell the new nurse who came to help that they had not called for help. (This happened about three times before they finally figured out what was going on.)

After resolving the potty passing out performance, the remainder of the family's visit to room 25 seemed to be consumed with discussions about my color as it slowly came back from ashen to a rosy hue. (I know the shades because as I told you earlier, the bed faced the only mirror in the room!) Bruce seemed to stay somewhat ashen up until the time that he left for home close to 10. He did stay long enough to witness me go to the bathroom again...this time without passing out. From that point on, I would be going to the bathroom every 1.5 to 2 hours around the clock. (So much for sleep.)

One of the most important things to do when faced with a situation like this cancer is to get your head on straight. I could panic. I could cry. I could wail and scream at how unfair life is. I could even get really high up on my self-pity pot and point fingers at God. I believe that none of those choices are the right direction to go, however. I believe that the secret to improvement and progress through the process lies in celebrating the small victories! I believe in the joy in life, and finding the joy, wonder, encouragement, and humor in every circumstance that I can.

With this attitude, I can honestly tell you what a wonderful week I have had. There have been so many small victories...so many triumphs. They have all been rewarded with continuing good news. I had many opportunities to laugh and enjoy life all week long.

At the beginning of this post, I told you that the two main lessons were going to the bathroom and suction related. You now know about that first trip to the potty. Tomorrow, I will fill you in on some amusing times in the hospital, and more than you ever wanted to know about suction bags.

15
Drainage Tubes and Drama

Many beautiful events in life involve discomfort and/or pain. The one that comes quickest to mind is giving birth. (Then comes the pain of raising the child/children into worthwhile adults; but that is more emotional than physical . . . usually . . . but that is another story!) With natural child birth, there is the pain of the actual labor . . . passing a watermelon sized person through a quarter sized hole . . . does take some fortitude . . . and these days, some drugs. With a C-section, there is a different type of pain . . . but still drugs.

However birth is done, the afterbirth must come out. Because the body is built the way it is, gravity helps (as do the natural openings in the body).

After other internal surgeries, other waste products must also come out. Gravity is not as helpful in many of these cases, and with the removal of a breast, there are no natural openings for the waste products of the breast to drain from. So, man invented the drain tubes.

From an analytical perspective, the drain tube is wonderful in its simplicity. A section of tube is left inside of the body with connection to another tube outside of the body and a bulb devise on the end of that tube that can create a suction to draw waste products from the body. I pictured in my mind the internal tubing being like a soaker hose for the garden, but in reverse. My home healthcare nurse confirmed today that I have a pretty good comparative image of how the system works.

One of the first things that I learned upon reaching room 25 was that I now had two drain tubes extruding from my body. One was above where my breast used to be, the other below. Their main purpose is to take up the slack from where the lymph nodes were removed while my body grows new pathways to dispose of the fluids that the now missing lymph nodes once handled. I knew that I would have them because I had done my internet research and seen garments that have pockets to place the suction bulb into, and the surgeon had told me. What I didn't know, and no one told me, was that I was responsible for showing up with any of these specialized garments that I chose to use, or work up whatever system I could come up with for dealing with them. Otherwise, I could carry them or they could dangle . . . which I quickly discovered was NOT a pleasant experience . . . especially when they were full of fluid.

After the passing out on the potty incident, Bruce informed me that he was grading my recovery process and that so far, I was failing. This did not make me very happy, being the teacher that I am, and he refused to provide me with a syllabus or rubric that would spell out for me what the criteria was for success, so I ended up stumbling through my recovery like many kids stumble through their classes . . . without a clue how to succeed.

As I told you before, Bruce did see me make it to the potty once without passing out before he left the night after the surgery. What I didn't tell you was that I learned on that occasion that it is very important to not forget that the drain tubes were hanging from your body. (I learned a couple of other important lessons at that time too.)

My second trip to the restroom, I decided to plan a bit ahead. I did much mental prepping, and requested my wonderful morphine (you may still hurt, but you really don't care) be given to me about 20 minutes before my trip rather than waiting to see if I would need it afterwards as I had done the first time. Then, about 10 minutes before I felt like it might be too late for my bladder, I called for the nurse. (I really was tethered to the bed by all sorts of devices: EKG equipment, blood pressure cuff, IV, nasal oxygen tubing, and oxygen saturation finger cuff. All of these had to be disconnected prior to my travelling the 10 feet to relieve myself.)

Since I now knew that my performance was being graded, I was determined to be a fast learner. Everything was disconnected; nurse on my right, Bruce on my left. All I had forgotten as I stood up was the two (very full) drainage bags that were attached to my fresh wounds. When they fell from the bed to the end of their tethers, I nearly failed again! I was glad that I had already had my morphine and it had had a chance to take effect.

(Note to self: Always request that the nurse empty the drainage bags BEFORE making the trip to the restroom…just in case they fall again.) When they fell, and I let a naughty word or two escape my lips, Bruce looked me in the eyes and said, "Babe, what did you want to do that for? Looks like that had to hurt. Why don't you carry them next time?" (At least he made me laugh!)

From that point forward, the drainage bags continued to be a source of both frustration and fascination from me. I would continue to drop them on occasion and swear to myself that I would not forget them again. I was mesmerized by the (what I found out later) blood clots running through the tube of number 2. They formed dark magenta spirals through the tube that other drainage would continue to flow around. The scientific part of my mind drew interesting correlations with other spirals that occur in nature; the double helix, curly hair, and other things such as springs and twining tree trunks. One thing is certain; I was never bored by them.

On Monday when I arrived in room 25, my wonderful nursing staff told me to rest and enjoy as much as I could because on Tuesday, the work would start. They were not joking.

As Monday rolled into Tuesday with my every 2 hour trips to the bathroom, as the nurse disconnected me for my 5am trip to relief, she told me that soon, I would not be disconnected, but would travel with my equipment still attached. Around 7 am, I was relieved of the nasal oxygen tubes and the EKG leads. Blood pressure cuff and finger tether were removed a short while later. I also conned the nurse into leaving the IV unplugged long enough to put on my pajama top and changing out of the breezy gown. (I think that she agreed because I had already managed to change out of my now smelly hot pink underpants and into my pajama bottoms…no more free show for passers by!)

I had several visitors on Tuesday. Each member of my surgical team came by at one point or another to let me know that their prayers were with me and to wish me well in the rest of my battle. Mother and Zoe came for most of the day. (Bruce was back at work…in a class to recertify.) And one of the teachers I work with surprised me pleasantly at lunch with a visit. An arm sling was ordered for my left arm so that I could walk without causing fluid to accumulate in my arm and create a complication called lymphedema. (If you want to gross yourself out, look it up on Google images!) I was told to get up and move as much as possible. I tend to do as I am told when it seems appropriate.

Whenever I was awake and up to it, I took my IV stand in my right hand, left arm in a sling with drainage bulbs in hand, and headed out to walk the halls of the hospital. (Now that I was out of my room, I was especially glad that I had brought some real jammies rather than relying on a hospital gown. I would have been one hand short!)

Shortly after Mother and Zoe left for lunch, and I had drunk my chicken broth (my nurse was not too fond of working quickly and had not passed on the orders for REAL food to the kitchen yet even though the doctor issued them at 9am), I had time for a quick nap. I was not expecting anyone to come back in until much later in the afternoon since Bruce was still in his class and Mom and Zoe were going to be running errands after they ate. The time was right, so I snuggled in for a snooze.

Immediately upon waking up, I, of course, went to the restroom. As I was coming back out, I heard an alarm of some sort going off in the hall. It was followed by an announcement, "Ladies and Gentlemen, a fire has been detected in the building. Please proceed in an orderly manner to the nearest exit."

I froze in place, thinking, "You've got to be kidding me!"

Since the alarm was continuing to go off and the announcement played again, I put on my sling, stuck my cell phone and Kindle into it along with my left arm, and grabbed my IV stand. As I unplugged my IV stand, and new voice spoke over the recorded announcement and stated that this was a false alarm and please ignore the sirens . . . that they were working on it and would fix it as quickly as possible.

Laughing to myself in disbelief, I removed my Kindle from my sling and walked down to the nurse's station to try and find out which of the voices to believe. It turns out that a visitor to the hospital had brought her 4-5 year old son with her. She left him unattended in the secondary lobby at the end of my hall. He found the fire alarm and did what curious young boys who are left to their own devices do . . . he pulled the handle. Several of the nurses were very angry with the young mother for yelling at the boy in her embarrassment and felt that someone should have been yelling at the young mother for her lack of parenting and attention to her child.

By the time Bruce made it to the hospital, Zoe and Mother were back. Zoe was bragging to her daddy about my progress in healing and asking him what grade I had for the day. He told her that only what he sees me do with his own eyes counts, and that if I want a good grade, I need to show him myself. I did not mind. I realize that he was, in his gentle and teasing way, providing me with a way to push myself to get better and come home. It seems that he doesn't sleep well when I am away any more than I can sleep when he is away. After snuggling together for 22 years, our bed gets lonely whenever one of us is using it alone. We were both relieved when Dr. G2, my surgeon, came back by and stated that he was fairly certain that he would be releasing me the next morning.

With that knowledge, I slept much better the second night. I only requested the morphine twice, and woke the next day fresh and happy in the knowledge that I would be home before Bruce got done with his last day of recertification classes.

16
Tube Troubles and Coming Events

Yesterday, we discussed some of the fun of having drainage bags. There are several challenges that go along with them too. Possibly the most challenging aspect came to light sometime around the day after my release from the hospital.

After surgery, your body goes through an adjustment period. As the swelling shrinks, other things began to become obvious . . . for example; I am estimating that I have 2-4 feet of tubing buried under my skin from each of the drainage set-ups. This may not sound like a very bad deal since they are buried under the skin, but it creates an interesting map of hills and valleys in an area where there once sat one mountain. The largest gathering of the tubes seems to lie under my arm. (Let's just say that showing up naked is not what it once was . . . not bad as long as I don't lift my arm.) It feels (from my perspective) as if someone has planted an upwardly rising river that wants to overflow the banks of my bodily boundaries. It becomes more obvious each day, and I am ready to kiss the feet of the doctor who removes this uncomfortable mass from its bulging territory under my arm... It may well be the most uncomfortable experience I have ever had. The bonus is that I will get an opportunity to repeat this fun when I have the rebuild in 6 months or so. (Yee-haw...can hardly wait!)

Another fun piece of trivia about this experience is that I have developed seromas. Seromas are (according to Dr. G2)areas where the lymph fluid tries to escape in an unusual manner. This is the most common post-surgical complication after any breast surgery with approximately 80% of women getting to experience the joy. Sometimes, they form deep within the breast where the tissues have been removed. In my case, they appear as varying sized blood blisters on the surface of where my breast once was, but very near the healing scar areas. Most are small and lie along the incision lines. I have one very large one that sits next to my already abused nipple. (Thank God for bandages which hide the mess!) The last bit of fun with Seromas is that they tend to break and leak. Remember when you just had the baby and your milk would let down…similar situation/sensation…just with a bloody mess leaking out rather than that watery milk.

Bruce took off work today so that he could accompany me to my first oncology appointment and hear the answer to the burning question, "What next?"

First, the pathology results from the mastectomy . . . all margins were completely clear of cancer. This means that they got all of the original cancer. Ten lymph nodes were removed, and four of them were 'infected' with the cancer cells. Finally, there was a 'thread' of the cancer going from one of the lymph nodes into the muscle wall of my chest in the diaphragm area. In spite of the bad news, with the completely clear margins, Dr. K1 stated that my cancer WAS Stage III due to the size of the tumors, the number of lymph nodes involved, and the aggressive speed with which it reared its ugly head.

Bruce was very relieved to hear Dr. K1 state several times that the coming chemo and radiation followed by hormone therapy are measures to prevent recurrence of the cancer in the same area, or from a metastasis of the cancer to other organs. So, my 'preventative' chemo will begin on September 2. I will receive 4 rounds of the first medication, followed by 3 rounds of the second medication, followed by 6-7 weeks of daily radiation. (That is the one that is potentially tricky schedule wise…)

While his presentation was geared to 'preventative', it was obvious to us that he has never received the results of the bone scan, and he had missed the muscle wall involvement in the initial report. Now that he is aware of them, he is requesting the bone scan results and will either keep the same program, or make changes as appropriate with the new information.

Whether it is, or it was, we are geared up for the continuing fight and ready to get the show on the road. Now, if I can just get Dr. G2 to remove these stupid tubes on Wednesday, I will be a very happy camper….but not until the tubes are OUT!!!

17
Holey Tube Removal, Batman!

Yesterday was the first of two exchange days held in our school district. In preparation, I did something for the first time in my life that most women have experienced, but I had never had the occasion to . . . I had to learn how to stuff my bra. It took a couple of tries before I was satisfied that they were close to the same size, although the false one was rather perky compared to the sag on my real one.

I reported to work with everyone else and was surprised to find that they were surprised to see me there even though I had assured them that I would come. I felt very welcome, and although I allowed myself some physical accommodations in order to function, I did not feel that there was anyone who resented those special accommodations. The team I was assigned to was wonderful, and we got much done. It was great to see everyone from the English department. I was, however, totally exhausted by the time I got home.

My home healthcare nurse was due to come over at 4:30 to redress my surgical site, so I rushed home and jumped into the shower at 4:15. When I got out, I knew that I was so tired that I would not go anywhere for the rest of the evening, so I dressed in my lounging jammies and got comfortable. After my nurse completed my check up and left, I sat down in my recliner and signed onto Facebook very briefly. One of my dear friends checked in on me through chat and asked how the day went. When I told her how tired I was, her response was, "so, rest." Deciding that she was very wise, I signed off and curled up under my Snuggie (Mother made it for me a couple of Christmases ago and I find it very comfortable and comforting after surgeries), and was asleep by 5:15 pm. I woke up just after 8 pm. (Guess I really was tired!)

49

Today was round two. Two of the best additions that have been made to our school library, where we have been meeting, are the reading areas with comfortable sofas, loveseats, and chairs. They are big and luxurious, and I chose to sit on one of the sofas today rather than in my desk chair. With my arm propped up on pillows, I was much more comfortable today and as a result have more energy this evening (although I am still quite tired).

I left during the meetings to go for my surgical follow up exam at 9:45 this morning. Having arrived and checked in at 9:30, I began to be concerned at 10:15 when 5 other patients who had arrived after me had been called back before me. I asked and was told that I was the next person in the cue. By 10:25, I was in the exam room and dressed in one of the fashionable, highly ventilated gowns, and waiting for the doctor.

By 11:25, the exam room had become very stuffy and I was beginning to seethe about still waiting to see the doctor for my 9:45 appointment. I knew that he was there because I had heard him many times in the rooms on either side of me. Finally, at 11:45, two hours after my appointment was scheduled, I opened the door and asked the nurses if I should simply get dressed and reschedule for a more convenient time. They again told me not to do that since I was the next patient up in the cue. A couple of minutes later, I heard the pharmaceutical rep who was standing at the nurse's station tell the doctor that he would come back later because there was a very irate patient in the exam room who had been waiting over an hour for her appointment. The doctor came in then, very contrite, and tried to explain that he was caught up with a patient who wanted to be treated for an illness that he did not have. I told him that I would probably forgive him if he would remove the 'dad-gummed tubes'. He assured me that he had planned to do that today.

I must admit at this point that I had over-estimated the length of the tubes that were burrowed under my skin, and which one went where. It turned out that the lower tube was the one that was zigzagged through my chest. It was only about 18 inches long. The other one, the upper one, was the one that was most driving me crazy. It had been spiraled under my arm...burrowing into my arm pit...and was only about 24 inches long. He removed both with little effort on the part of either of us. Since everything still feels like a foot that has gone to sleep (only not exactly a foot), there was no pain. The nurse, however, did make me laugh with the look of pain that came over her face as she watched each tube being removed. She also winced as Dr. G2 began to remove each of the 20 staples from the incision. She really became uncomfortable when he handed the tool over to her and told her to get the rest while he went to get a special tool for the one he could not reach up under my arm. I finally took pity on her and told her that I had little to no feeling where she was working and that she would not hurt me. She seemed to relax then.

Dr. G2 was concerned about the seromas, but knew that time was the only real treatment that we can use for them. He put 3 nurses to work wrapping up the incision site again, beginning with a Betadyne bath for the whole thing. It became rather funny when they tried to place the Betadyne in the deep recess under my arm where they had trouble removing that one deep-set staple. The closest sensation that I can use to explain what I experienced when they pressed medicine in there is a tickling sensation . . . which is unusual since I am not normally ticklish under my arms. They would press and I would squirm. (Sometimes words are not adequate to describe sensations, and I found my attempted explanations falling short.) We did share a few laughs over my reactions though!

After the Betadyne, the nurse placed a lightweight, flexible mesh of some sort, and the group appeared to be painting it on somehow. They then began with layers, and layers, upon layers and layers of gauze and padding. I finally asked the nurse if she was just going to build me a new prosthesis right then, and complained that I would need to remove the stuffing from my bra or be lopsided the other way!

Because of the delay, lunch was hurried, but I did take the time to run by the house and take a pain pill (just in case). Before going to my afternoon meetings, I had a thought . . . and, as is the case with many of my thoughts, I told Zoe. I said, "Hey, Zoe. Do you realize that your mother is now a doubly holey woman?"

Her response was, "Ha, ha. Very funny. I get it Mom."

18
Reflections on Healing

God has a sense of humor.

I have wondered every day while I have this neuropathy why the home healthcare nurses always ask me about my pain levels. It has been a puzzlement since all I have ever been able to tell them is that the sensation is like a foot that has gone to sleep . . . although in the wrong place.

About 4 o'clock this morning, I woke up (in more ways than one) to understanding. It seems that as the nerves begin to knit and feeling returns, the first and most prominent sensation is pain. The feeling that woke me at 4 am was that of having the hairs of my underarm being pulled slowly out by the root! Yikes!

On a positive note, as the seromas are healing across the nipple that the surgeon insisted on saving, they are leaving behind new, pink, fresh skin. This skin has some feeling . . . a light tingling, slight stinging sensation . . . much as any blister that pops and loses its protective dead skin feels. While the surgical sight is kept tightly 'under wraps' in an effort to maintain moisture in the skin, the healing of the places where the tubes resided under my skin are very noticeable and the areas of the greatest sensation. Those which are under my arm can still be traced as if the 24 inches of tubing were still present although all that tubing was removed last Wednesday. It does create some interesting lines under my clothing.

As with any wound healing, there is itching. This may prove challenging next week when I return to work. There is just no nice way to scratch an itch in a place that is as prominent as high up on the front of your ribcage! Here at home, I have managed to get some relief from the itching by doing the 'referred' itch scratch. In other words, when the left side itches, I scratch on the right side in the same place. (This is an old trick that has been taught to kids with broken bones for generations. It allows relief from the itch without causing additional wounds to the area that is healing.)

With cancer, you need to address the healing of not only the body, but the mind. In keeping with my so far successful campaign to use laughter as my number one medicine, I have been reading uplifting stories from other cancer survivors. My current book, Chicken Soup for the Cancer Survivor's Soul, is one that was recommended to me by Vera' when she was going through her treatments. My favorite story so far is the one written about the young woman's first trip for a mammogram. It seems that after she was strapped into the machine and the test was just started, the machine caught on fire! Her account shows the humor and reality that I can appreciate! I laughed so hard, and bookmarked it in my kindle so that I could read it to Bruce when he came home. (I do wonder though if she ever went back for another mammogram after the first one!)

In my reflections over this experience, I think often about the mammogram. Ladies, I believe that if men were required to use this same method for regular checks for testicular cancer, we would be gifted very quickly with a more comfortable way to check and maintain our good health. (I just can't imagine most men undergoing what we undergo more than once without inventing a better way to check for cancer.)

As I sit here enjoying (NOT) the sensation of underarm hair in a death grip, I believe that losing my hair to chemo will have its benefits; saving a fortune on shampoo, no longer needing to shave legs and pits, and best of all…no need to wax the upper lip and chin that seem to be taking on the hair that has left the legs as I have gotten older. Nearly any situation can have a positive side if you just look at it from the right direction. Now, if you will please excuse me….I need to go scratch an itch!

19
Planning Ahead and Blessings

It has been brought to my attention that some of you may be uncomfortable with my 'tell all' style of writing about this experience, but I am writing about all of the things that everyone who is familiar with the trials and tribulations of breast cancer fails to tell you to expect. To me, it would have been natural and normal to warn a breast surgery patient to be prepared for the seromas, for example, since they afflict 80-90% of all breast surgery patients. However, not only was I not prepared or warned about them, my home healthcare nurses did not know what they were until I found the information online and they verified it with the surgeon. Now that they are being treated, they are behaving much better and I appear to be up in the 'super healing' category.

Having started back to work on in-service this week in preparation for getting students next week, I have been out of the house much more and participating. Like I have told my coworkers who have asked, I could be uncomfortable at home, or I can be uncomfortable at work and accomplishing something . . . I choose to accomplish something. When I put it that way, they seem to understand my decisions. So many people seem to think that since I am officially an 'amputee' now, I should take a great deal of time and take things easy. I am managing to take it easy while accomplishing something. I must admit though that when I get home, my tired is hanging out!

At this time, the oncologist has told us that I will lose all of my hair within 7-10 days of starting the chemo. He says that with this particular medication it happens like clockwork. After discussing it with Bruce, our plan is to have the first round of chemo on September 2, and then find a hairdresser who will cut off my hair and shave my head. This should allow me to donate the hair, and forestall the potential plumbing problems that would be brought on by having 14 or more inches of very thick hair falling off in the shower. I had grown it out to donate, so this is a good plan for me. I had originally planned to just do it myself, but when I told Bruce, he suggested that I find a hairdresser who was willing to send it off for me.

My home healthcare nurse called her friend (who is a cosmetologist in a local hair salon) to see if she would be willing to take it down to bald for me and send in the donation. She is, and she will do the deed either on the 2nd or 3rd. I have also already told my boss (who is follicle-ly challenged) that when we return from Labor Day, I will show him what bald is supposed to look like!

With Bruce by my side, I am considering myself to be so very blessed! I had a first husband who would not speak to me or look at me for 2 weeks after I got a really cute haircut many years ago. When he finally spoke to me, it was to tell me that I was 'not allowed' to ever cut my hair again without his express permission. That was the first husband. Bruce is my last husband.

When I chose to go bald with my dear friend Vera' when her metastatic breast cancer recurred in 2006, Bruce not only supported my decision, he stood by with the camera taking pictures. He has been there for me through 2 C-sections, a hysterectomy, a spontaneous miscarriage, knee surgery, a gallbladder removal, and now with breast cancer and subsequent mastectomy. Knowing that things look pretty ugly right now, I asked him the other day if he was at all repulsed…his reply was that I still look the same on the inside. He is truly the best husband I could ever ask for, and I don't half deserve him!

Well, the pain is setting in again. The nurses tell me that the pain is a good sign…that it means that I will get to keep what little I have left of the breast because the pain indicates that healing is happening. I am glad that I am seeing the surgeon again tomorrow so that I can ask him about switching around the pain medications so that I can spend less time hurting and more time working. I am highly allergic to hydrocodone which is what is typically prescribed post-surgery, so they simply put me on prescription strength Tylenol. It was sufficient when I was numb with the neuropathy, but it is not convincing me that it does anything anymore. Maybe he will let me add some Advil in between the 3 daily doses of Tylenol to take the edge off! I guess I will find out tomorrow!

Have a great tonight and a wonderful tomorrow. (I plan to!)

20
Back to Work and Other Adventures

This was back to school week for teachers here in Fort Stockton. We had meetings, district- wide, most days. Some days, we were campus only. Others, we were department only. But, the real work and preparation for the coming school year was done this week. It was also my first week back to work for 40 hours with no napping time.

As I set out to 'get the job done' this week, most folks in the district were wonderfully supportive of me and my efforts to keep as high a level of normalcy as possible while dealing with cancer. The staff at the middle school where we held most of our meetings was wonderful about bringing me a "special" chair to sit in that had a comfortable seat, padded back, and armrests (which are still vitally important)! We would spend long hours seated in the cafeteria while various speakers went over important points and motivational information. Anyone who has ever attended an in-service for teaching could probably sing line and verse of these to you without even knowing the topics under discussion. Two of the days were devoted to preparation of ways to teach for success on the 'new and improved' state assessment here in Texas.

I found myself increasingly tired by the end of the week. On Wednesday, I left the meetings for another follow up with my surgeon to check on my progress with healing. While in his office, his nurse worked me over with Betadyne, and hydrogen peroxide to try and make sure that the dead tissue from the burst seromas was sloughing off and allowing the new skin from underneath to grow back. By the end of the ordeal, I felt like I had undergone some sort of very aerobic workout for an extended period. I managed to grab a lunch on the go, however, and make it back to the meetings in time to snag a decent parking place.

The surgeon decided to conduct an experiment with my bandages that proved to be . . . interesting.

Having been bandaged for over 2 weeks, the tape has decided that it needs to just fuse with the skin of my chest, abdomen, and underarm. When the nurse was removing it to work me over with the Betadyne and hydrogen peroxide bath, it was sticking so badly that it was taking my skin off with it when she would remove it. After attempting to just rip off a piece where my pectoral muscle attaches to my underarm and having it refuse to come off, she grabbed the tape softening wipes, which are basically just acetone, and soaked it off. When she applied it to the area where the tape was stuck most strongly, I discovered two things. (1) The skin underneath the tape had torn where she was trying to rip off the tape, and (2) I have gotten back much more feeling than I had realized (or really wanted at this point in time).

When the doctor came in and inspected his handiwork and my healing, we discussed the problem with the tape. He then formulated a plan to apply new bandages without tape. He explained his plan and the nurse thought that she understood.

After 30 minutes of bathing, swabbing, and what felt like a general assault (which I joked my way through rather than screaming), the plan for bandaging was put into effect. Neosporin was painted on. Light weave mesh was placed over that. Thin Teflon bandages were placed next, and followed by a thick padding. On top of all this, the nurse loosely piled wads of gauze. Then the tapeless part of the plan was implemented. While I held the wads of padding in place, the nurse took a tape measure and measured me from armpit to waist.

If you have ever had occasion to use a finger cover, then you can imagine the stuff that was cut to fit. This was the same stretchy stuff, only open at both ends, and slightly wider than a finger cuff. (I am quite a bit wider than a finger cuff, so I knew that things were about to get interesting.)

The plan was for the nurse to stretch this new cuff over my head and arms while I held onto the wads of bandaging, keeping it all in place, as she fitted the finger sleeve on me like a tube-top. (It was a very good thing that the mesh was stretchy!) With much giggling on both of our parts (the nurse at the station kept popping in to see what was going on because she felt left out with all of the laughing), we managed . . . somehow . . . to get the stretchy-mesh in place and reposition the bandages with both of my arms on the outside.

We had a new problem . . . every time the nurse let go of the mesh that was now holding the bandages in place, it rapidly rolled up on both ends to the middle and dropped out wads of gauze. Obviously, I was not going to be able to go back to work with a nurse attached to me, no shirt on, and clouds of gauze drifting lazily out of the new contraption. We decided that we needed to find a better means of holding the ends down than using the nurse. What to do? What to do?

Holding on to the wads and pads and (as best I could) the wrap, the nurse left me to grab my mastectomy bra.

For those of you who don't know, a mastectomy bra is one that has pockets to allow for 'stuffing' to be placed inside of one pocket to provide the illusion of having matching breasts. (I knew girls in high school who would have loved to know about this contraption!) It has pockets on both sides to allow the wearer to stuff either side, or both, and provide the illusion of symmetry. (Many people become uncomfortable visually when they see a person resembling a Cyclops rather than a two breasted woman.) Mine had stuffing added to the left cup. I have needed at various times to adjust the amount of fiberfill in the pillow cushion that passes for a breast due to the amount of bandaging provided by the various nurses that have dressed my surgical wounds. Sometimes it is more, sometimes less. This exercise was not going to allow me the time to pull out any of the stuffing due to the need for more hands to make this new contraption work!

Doing a quick transfer, the nurse handed me the bra in my left hand while I held on to the billowing clouds of wrappings with my right. She frantically grabbed for the rolls that were happening in each direction with the slightly larger than finger wrap tube-top that I was now wearing as I rapidly tried to put on both sleeves to fasten it in the front. We had decided to try to secure the rolling mess with the bra to keep the bandages contained. Again, as we went through this process amid shouts of laughter, the nurse in the hall, like a well-timed jack in the box, popped her head in to see if everything was alright.

We finally had everything contained . . . somewhat . . . with the bra. I immediately noticed that I was now about a DDD on my left side and a C-D on my right due to the billowing clouds of gauze under my fiberfill. Figuring that I could use my pillows and posture to hide the difference throughout the remainder of the workday, I put on my shirt and headed back to work.

The nice thing about fiberfill is that you can smash it down and around and flatten it out to some extent! I returned to work hoping that it would be enough.

Once back at work, I discovered that the new system had some drawbacks. Periodically, I would feel the bandages shift inside their holder. I would quietly get up and go to the restroom and while hidden in a stall, rearrange things. Also, every time I would sit down the bottom of the tube would roll up and leave a roll sitting just under my ribcage. Again, I would excuse myself to the restroom for an adjustment. I finally solved this by tucking the bottom of the tube into my pants. This left me with my pants up like Steve Urkel, but since I was wearing my shirt untucked, it covered my nerdy apparel.

Wednesday was probably the most difficult day with the new bandaging system. Because I had gone into the doctor, I would not be getting new bandages until after 5 pm on Thursday evening. That put me living with the new system for over 24 hours. It felt like I was constantly tucking, pulling, or heading to the restroom.

By the afternoon, I found another new issue . . . my bra was heading north on the left while gravity was pulling me south on the right! This added a new dimension to my restroom trips. The routine became lift, lower, reposition, lower, tuck, and walk with grace as I used my underarm pillow to push down on the padding and my right arm to lift up on the rest.

Wednesday evening, the only way I could change into my pajamas was to have my wonderful daughter, Zoe, help me by holding up the back of the tube while I positioned the front.

Sleep on Wednesday night was the real adventure. Every time I would move, wads of padding and stuffing would shuffle and shift and I would traipse into the bathroom, close the door, and turn on the light so that I could see to reposition the bandages and pull out the roll at the top of the tube. When I got up with Bruce on Thursday morning, there was a trail of gauze pieces on the floor leading from my side of the bed to the bathroom like the crumbs dropped by Hansel and Gretel as they wondered through the woods. I quickly collected the pieces and threw them in the trash.

I got up extra early on Thursday morning so that Bruce could help me unroll the tube while I put the bra on to attempt to hold it in place. On a positive note, I had lost enough of the stuffing that I did not need to remove any of the fiberfill from my prosthesis. I was back down to a C-D on the left side too.

Thursday we were working at the high school, so I was happy to be able to have Zoe with me. She made many trips with me to the restroom to help me adjust the rapidly dwindling supply of bandaging inside the tube. By the time we left for home and I was able to shower before the home healthcare nurses arrived, I had a semi-permanent impression of the mesh weave in my stomach and probably across my back. I can't remember the last time a shower felt so good!

Having made it successfully through the week, by Friday evening I was exhausted. I missed out on my Facebook time because as soon as I sat down in my recliner, I was lost. I stayed awake long enough to enjoy pizza with the family, but fell asleep soon afterwards. I woke at 10 and headed to bed. Bruce and Zoe had quietly been working on the things that needed to be done around the house while I slept on, oblivious to what was happening around me. In fact, Bruce has declared today to be my day of rest in preparing for the kids to be in class next week. He has taken Zoe and the two are braving tax free shopping for school supplies, and then buying the groceries. How lucky I am to have the family that I do!

21
Updates on Healing

I have survived my first week back with students!

Monday was hard. I gave the standard talk to each of my classes in turn. They were mostly respectful and polite. I began by explaining to them that we don't always get to choose our journeys in life . . . that sometimes we are handed journeys that we must work our way through. One such journey that we will be taking together this year is learning enough to be able to be successful on the new state assessments. Another journey that they will be taking with me is the fact that I was diagnosed with cancer this summer.

At this point, the students asked very intelligent questions which I answered to the best of my ability. We discussed the fact that I would be out periodically having chemo treatments, and the fact that not all substitute teachers followed the lesson plans. We left the class with the understanding that they, the students, would need to step up and help the substitutes to keep us all on track so that we could enjoy a productive year and meet our educational goals. They agreed to help me make that happen.

After school dismissed for the day, I rushed home on Monday for my shower before my home healthcare nurse arrived to change my bandages. She arrived and we took care of business. The nurse could tell that I was in some pain (my blood pressure tends to tell all), and we redressed my surgical wounds. I then camped out in my easy chair with the intent of playing on Facebook.

Bruce got home just as the nurse was leaving. He fed me leftover ribs that he had cooked out on the grill the night before. I ate them, and then set up my computer to play.

I tried to play my games. I thought about how relaxed playing my games makes me feel. That was about as far as I got. I was asleep in my recliner by 7:45.

When the news was winding down at about 10:25, Bruce attempted to wake me to get me to go sleep in our bed. He ended up needing to half-way carry me down the hall to our room where I changed into my pajamas (pretty much in my sleep) and laid down to continue sleeping. I slept through to Tuesday morning. I was just awake enough when I lay down to hear him tell me that our daughter said to tell me good night.

For most of this week, I have been going to bed before my eleven year old. I get up before her too, but I have missed the nightly ritual of telling her 5-10 times that it is time for her to get to bed and go to sleep. (Funny how you can miss those little battles.) Bruce has been taking the lead in getting her into bed and ready for school the next day . . . at least each night.

My days have been filled with laughter and learning. I seem to have made the lucky draw this year with the most wonderful students! During our lesson on Thursday, one of them announced a foolish mistake that he had made on his grammar journal. It seems that where the example in the power point said for him to write his name (and used 'student name' in the example), he wrote 'student name' on his paper. We all laughed together, and I asked them if they knew how to make a blonde laugh on Friday. When they didn't know, I told them to tell her a joke on Wednesday. (Some of them had to have others explain it to them, and we laughed together about that.) I then pointed out to them that I am a blonde. I went on to tell them that I will develop a case of dyslexia next week and that my blonde jokes would become 'bald' jokes.

We had excellent discussions, and students were able to tell me at the end of each class many on topic things that they had learned during each lesson. This made me a very happy teacher! Our week ended with many of the students telling me that they can't wait for Monday so that they can see what they have to learn then! Strangely, I believed most of them.

My home healthcare nurse has expressed that she is very pleased with my healing progress. Each evening, I have had better color, and about ¼ inch of shiny new pink skin where I had bruising and blisters before. All of the seromas have burst and most of them have peeled leaving much healthier new skin behind. My pain levels have also gone down drastically as the week has progressed. I can walk quite well (I walked 10.4 miles, according to my pedometer, in class on Wednesday), but I tend to become tired and sore if I stand without walking for extended periods of time. In addition to the success walking, I have begun stretching and am nearly able to touch my thumbs behind my back when I do. I am able to use both arms to wash, brush, and style my hair.

The pain has gotten much better. We discovered on Wednesday that while the nurses had been putting bandages on while I was lying down, when I would sit up, the 'tucked-hole' under my arm (which was where I was experiencing the most pain) was becoming exposed. It seems that the hole moves when I sit up. Since this discovery, we have been applying the front of the bandage, and then having me sit up to apply the rest. This has kept the hole covered. Since the majority of my pain was associated with that hole, having it well covered has allowed me much greater comfort. Today was mostly pain free, except when I got hot.

The major sensation today occurred between 3rd and 4th period. (Thankfully, it hit between classes.) I developed a MAJOR itch deep inside the wound. When the itching started, I thought I might come unhinged! I squeaked and squawked, and finally ran to the restroom where I could secretly rub the itch through the bandages for a minute or two. By the time the tardy bell rang, I was back in class and comfortable again.

Tomorrow may be a challenge for me. Each teacher is required to serve 3 hours working at the concession stand. I am scheduled to work from 1-4. When I texted my wonderful husband, he texted back that he will be there working it with me! I know that he wants to be sure that I don't overdo and set the healing back. (I am still unable to lift more than my purse with my left arm, and there is also that standing still issue.) He has been my rock and strength throughout this ordeal, and I feel truly blessed to have him in my life!

22
As Chemo Approaches

This week has been one of the most radical rollercoaster rides so far in dealing with this mutiny of my body called cancer. With my first chemo treatment looming on the horizon this Friday, and the farewell to my long blonde locks creeping ever nearer, I have been rather anxious about just what all is about to happen within my system.

Feeling came back suddenly to the nipple area of my breast on Saturday evening. I can feel the bandages, and the pressure from the bra and pillow prosthesis, and it drives me crazy!!! When it first came up, like a freight train determined to get my attention, my first thought was to strip down and run around the house topless. I next thought about coming up with some sort of old Star Trek costume where I covered up my one breast and just left the bandages covering the other side. (Being practical, I decided to just adjust and try to get used to the new sensations.) After today, I have decided to use my summer tops with their shelf bras as undershirts, and just stick my pillow prosthesis in and hope it doesn't wonder around too much during the day.

I have had many hours to think, plan, laugh, and worry. My greatest fears at this point in time have to do with staying on schedule with my coming chemo treatments. Today, one fear was put to rest.

In the healing from my surgery, the home healthcare nurses have been worried about an area on what is left of my breast that still weeps, and varies in color from light green to white (depending on when I have showered, and scrubbed the healing tissues). Because of these worries, they asked me to visit with my surgeon again this afternoon.

Dr. G2 came into the exam room, and after removing the bandages, he was very careful to tell me and point out all of the areas where the skin tissues are alive and doing well. As is his typical fashion, he stressed the positive. What he does not say comes across loud and clear. He told me that the area under the white was where one of the larger of the 3 tumors had been located. He feels that there is a good chance that the weepy light green to white skin is no longer living tissue. I am still on track to start the chemo on Friday. In fact, he stated that if my oncologist has any doubts about starting the chemo to have him call Dr. G2. There is a good probability, however, that at some point in the near future, Dr. G2 will need to go back in and remove the questionable area so that I am left with good skin tissue once again.

With this idea in mind, he invited me to come back, yet again, in two weeks. At that time, he will look again at the progress of my healing and determine if it will be necessary to go back and cut out the area and stitch it back to a healthier state of healing. He will only do this after seeing the area and consulting with my oncologist to determine the best time within my treatment schedule to make such a move. (The chemo will cause problems with my blood production and only after I begin will we know how much the chemo will affect me.) Meanwhile, I am still on schedule to start the lifesaving process of destroying the cancer. It is this scheduling that has had me so concerned for the past few days. I feel that it is vital that I start this process and get busy with the fight!

Yesterday morning, I discovered that somewhere among my coworkers I have a wonderful friend and guardian angel. I just don't have any clue about who the person is to thank. In my box at work, I found a beautiful worry stone. It is clear acrylic, sized just right to hold in my hand, with a beautiful, three-dimensional pink cancer ribbon centered in the stone. As I work and silently pray that all goes according to plan, I have been finding comfort in rubbing the smooth surface of the beautiful stone. (I just wish I knew who to thank for the very thoughtful, very helpful gift.)

Between the gift and the visit with Dr. G2, I am feeling much more positive and have my happy attitude back. I am ready, and have been ready for a while, to start actively fighting this rebellion.

In the much too much time I have to think about things, I find myself wondering how women who don't have the perineural involvement in their breast cancer can come to terms mentally with the fact that they have cancer. The pain caused by this involvement is what we feel brought the cancer to our attention and possibly saved my life. It is what made the cancer hurt. 92% of all breast cancer patients do not have perineural involvement. Having experienced the pain has made me more aware of the cancer, and even though I no longer have the pain after the mastectomy, I remember having it and know that it was real. Aside from that experience, I feel fine . . . much as I did before the surgery. Feeling fine, yet knowing that I have a life threatening disease going on is very surreal to me. It causes me to question if all of this is real. Knowing that I feel that way, I wonder how hard it must be for the typical cancer patient to willingly walk into treatment when they know that they will not feel fine after they start that treatment. It is a paradox in my mind.

On Sunday, I found a wonderful new song by Martina McBride. I do not plan to listen to it again anytime soon because it affected me so strongly. It is called "I'm Gonna Love You Through It". It is a song about breast cancer survivors. In the video, the song is broken up by many survivors talking about how very much the support of their friends, family, and loved ones meant in their recovery and ability to survive and beat cancer. I cried because I don't know if I can ever fully express to you how very much your prayers, love, and care have meant to me and are continuing to mean to me as I am approaching this 'fight for my life'. In looking at all that is going on (and thinking [too much] about everything) I feel that your gifts of prayer and care are gifts of life to me and possibly the most vitally important part of my recovery. You cannot possibly imagine how very much your support means to me during this time. I thank you with all of my heart and soul. Your comments on my notes, your private messages to me, your clicking 'like' on what I have written, your silent prayers...every single one of you are my angels and I feel so very, overwhelmingly blessed because of YOU.

God bless you all. I will continue to keep you informed of what is happening as I am able.

23
Keeping Things in Balance

Lately, I have been remembering fondly a time long, long ago. It was the spring after I turned 17. My older sister, Stacey, was 18 and a senior in High School, so I would have been a sophomore. The preceding Thanksgiving we had learned to ski at Buttermilk Mountain in Aspen, Colorado where I was the first person admitted to the Aspen Emergency room during that ski season. I had, newbie skier that I was, sprained my right knee. Given that experience, on this particular ski trip, I was the cautious one in the group.

Our family had travelled to Sipapu Ski Resort in New Mexico. We met up with another family from Lubbock while there, and there were two teen-aged boys in their party. We all decided to make our trips down the mountain as a foursome, with the teenagers sticking together.

The trails in Sipapu were awesome. Many of them were coated with 3 feet of fresh powder that no other skier had travelled down. Untouched snow.

We decided to make a bet about who in the foursome would fall down the least. I was very much in the lead since I was very cautious after my accident the preceding Fall (pun intended). Stacey and the boys accused me of skiing like a grandma. Never-the-less, I was very much winning our bet.

We had travelled down many unbroken trails, enjoying the feeling of being the first people to travel down them, and each of the others left bigger marks where they fell 2 or 3 times on each slope. By the second day, I still had a perfect record until my very public fall.

On the second day, with me so proud of having not fallen at all (and all of the others losing count of the number of times that they had fallen) we met up in the late afternoon at the base of the mountain, directly in front of the lodge, to discuss which trail to take next. That was when I fell. We were standing perfectly still (as happy skiers zipped to and fro) when for no apparent reason I fell on my face.

Another time that I had an issue with balance was when I was 16 and a student ambassador in Europe for the summer. We had travelled from Belgium to England on a night boat, crossing the English Channel. The seas that night were so rough that around sunset, for the first time in my life, I saw a person literally turn green and become ill. People had purchased tickets for the crossing that allowed them to sleep on the floor of the ship.

With the very rough seas, the ship would rise to the top of the crest and then drop, crashing to the bottom. Walking was taken by three of us as a carnival style challenge. On the up swell, while walking, it would feel as if our knees were trying to sink into our chests. When the ship would drop on the down, we would fly into the air to the point that our feet were not touching and we were flying. The trouble was, that with the people sleeping sickly on the deck, it was a challenge to touch down at the start of the next up swell without stepping on anyone. It became a game that three of us played all night while the rest of our group was in their births where the smell of the vomit was overwhelming!

After riding and playing all night, when we reached England, we immediately boarded a train and rode the swaying beast into London. I do not remember how long the ride took, but it took at least an hour or two. After the train, we boarded a bus which took us to our hotel.

Once we reached the hotel, while the teachers obtained our room keys, I stood still in the Lobby. That was when I discovered that as long as I was moving I was fine, but if I stood still, I needed to be propped up somewhere because if I stood in open space, I would quickly be hitting the floor. The inability to stand still in place without being propped up lasted until the following morning.

Since my surgery 30 days ago, I have noticed that I become tired very quickly, to the point of feeling like I will fall over, if I stand in one place. I have had days where I walked over ten miles in my classroom. (Most days,

I am walking over five miles in my classroom and around the school.) However, when I stand or sit in an unsupported chair, I am overwhelmed with fatigue to the point that I once again experience the feeling that I am about to simply fall over standing.

It has only taken me 30 days to realize the cause of this phenomenon. I am off balance. Because I am no longer symmetrical, I need to adjust my very center of balance in order to stand in place. The weight difference between my left and right sides is great enough to cause me to be unable to successfully stand still. Having finally figured this out for myself (another thing I wish someone had thought to mention might be an issue), I now understand why women pay to have a prosthetic breast fitted…it is a matter of balance!

At least you, my friends, always knew I was a bit off kilter. It just took me a while to figure it out!

24
Wardrobe Malfunction

Janet Jackson had the biggest recent notable accidental wardrobe malfunction and it was very public. Even if it had been in a less public arena, I feel certain that it would have been an embarrassment to her. Thankfully, the one I experienced today was not that bad, but it did have me laughing!

As the white skin on my surgical site peels away leaving the fresh pink skin in its place, I am experiencing more and more feeling. Things have gotten to the point where wearing my mastectomy bras is an uncomfortable experience. Because of this, I had decided that I would wear one of my summer tops with the shelf-bra as underwear and simply place my pillow prostheses inside. It was not until today that I decided that I had put together the right professional outfit to try it at school. With that goal in mind, this morning I took extra time to be sure that I had it filled with just the right amount of fiberfill to make it an even size with my one remaining breast . . . trying to achieve the most natural look that I can. I decided to wear a rather loud print blue top over all since I have discovered that the louder the print, the more it covers any size differences between my prosthetic pillow and my real breast. (During my off time, I have even been able to wear a loud print top around town without my prosthetic pillow and most people never realize that I am more flat-chested on my left side than my 19 year old son or my 11 year old daughter!)

Covered in this manner, I headed to work planning to tackle today's grammar lessons with the students easily and happily. (I have the world's best classes this year!) I headed into the school early so that I could have everything ready when the students arrived, and proceeded to take care of my normal morning 'running'.

I was floored when I checked my box and found another gift from my secret friend. Another teacher was standing close by and saw the gift too. She suggested jokingly that we use the cash that was contained in the card for lunch with me buying. (It appears that my secret friend knows exactly what I will be needing and when I will be needing it . . . as if either the secret friend has experienced all I am going through themselves, or with a close loved one.) In my surprise, I didn't think to check on things until I got back to my classroom.

Upon arriving back in my room, I glanced down at some papers and noticed that my pillow filler was poking its edge out from under my shirt, giving me the appearance of having a flesh colored growth where my cleavage used to be. Giggling with images of what might have happened if I had not noticed it before the students arrived; I headed for the bathroom to fix it.

The pillow put in another appearance at the start of 2nd period and again before 3rd. I became much more aware and worked to keep it down better after that.

By the time I got home for lunch, I was puzzling over the situation and trying to find a less time consuming way to handle the situation than constantly heading into the restroom to reposition things. As I was eating, the solution came to me. I finished eating, washed up and went to work.

Heading back to my bedroom to get the materials I needed, I lifted the print outer shirt, and the tank top portion of my summer shirt that was now acting as my undershirt. From this position, I took a safety pin and pinned my breast (the fake one) to my shelf bra, thus preventing it's reappearance for the afternoon. After that, I promptly forgot about my troubles from the morning.

Fiberfill has a way of travelling around when you are not paying attention to it. By the time I got home to shower before the home healthcare nurse came to change my bandages, my prosthetic pillow breast was sitting sideways in my shelf bra with the inside edge trying to put in an appearance out the top of my top! The pin held part of it down but not all. Next time, I plan to use two pins, but I will always keep loud print shirts handy! They camouflage things very well!

25
First Chemo and Hair

The much anticipated report on the first chemo is here and I am happy to say that so far the anticipation has been the worst part of the ordeal.

When we arrived for the appointment, Bruce (my wonderful, fantastic, fabulous husband) is my chemo buddy; we paid, signed forms and filled out papers as we were ushered back for blood tests. Since Bruce was wearing his GE Wind shirt, the lab lady struck up a conversation with him about wind turbines and solar power generation. She wanted to know everything with thoughts of putting her own power generation on her homestead. It was fine with me that they were visiting about all of this, but she was an animated talker. Bruce was standing in the doorway behind her as she talked and she kept turning to visit with him and jostling my arm while the needle was in for the pre chemo tests. Each time I was ready to say something to her about the pull of the needle; she would turn back my way and straighten things up again. When we finished up, she asked for our phone numbers so that she can get in touch with us over any further electrical generation questions she comes up with!

We were then sent back to the lobby for another wait. This one was short. We were ushered into the back for a weight check and then into an exam room for our visit with Dr. K1.

He checked my bandages and reviewed my treatments with me. Evidently, the new girl at the cardiologist's office was not inclined to look in my file and find my consent to release information and she would not share with the oncology offices the results of my tests. I signed another consent form with Dr. K1's nurse and Dr. K1 took a shortcut, calling Dr. G1 (the cardiologist) directly to get information on my results.

After we finished with the doctor, we were sent to scheduling where we set up the next chemo for Sept. 23, and went on to another waiting area until someone came to lead us through the maze to the chemo room.

The room where you receive chemo is large. It is sectioned into 3 separate administration areas with 8 patient chairs and 8 'buddy' chairs in each section. Restrooms are on each end. Coffee, juice, tea, and water are provided through large machines at the entrance. There is also a large selection of pastries on which to munch. For entertainment, portable DVD players are available with a large selection of movies. Windows stretch beside the administration area and look out onto an interior garden which had suffered a bit under the heat and lack of moisture from this record breaking summer drought.

We were shown around and ushered into the center area where we chose to sit beside the windows. We waited to see what would happen next. We did not have long to wait. My nurse came by just after I retrieved a snack from the bar and returned to my seat.

Before we could begin, the nurse had a large packet of information to go over with us. It listed the chemo cocktail du jour. Because the chemo that we start with is so strong, we had to be sure that the IV needle is threaded right. It was the worst part of the ordeal . . . getting the needle threaded right. Although well meaning, the nurse managed to blow out the backside of the vein twice before calling in a specialist who managed to thread it on the first try. (If they had been unable to get the needle threaded, I would have had to reschedule for another day so that we could try again.)

The importance of getting the needle threaded right with the type of chemo that has been prescribed for me is this; if the needle is not threaded right and any of the chemo gets out of the vein, it causes serious burns that can lead to permanent nerve damage. With only one arm that they can attempt (once you have had lymph nodes removed, that arm can never again be used to check blood pressure, or even draw blood), the IV needle MUST be set right. This is also why I have an appointment with another surgeon on September 12 to have a port installed.

A port sits just under the skin of your chest on your good side and has a lead line running directly into a vein so that all IVs can be injected through it without the need to run an IV line. It does not show under your clothes, and it can be left in place for future treatments and surgeries. Once we understood how it looks and how it functions, we wished that I had one installed years ago. It would have saved sooooo many failed IV insertion attempts!

After the nurse went over everything with us, we were on our own again as the saline dripped into my line. A beautiful older lady in a dew rag sat down across from us and proudly announced that she was there for her final chemo treatment. We celebrated together . . . her last treatment with my first.

The nurse sent in a lady to talk to me about my hair. They were afraid that I would be upset when I found out that I would lose all of my wonderful golden hair. I wish I had a photo of her face when I explained to her that I have been bald before! We explained that we were planning to do the pre-emptive head shave and donation of the hair. She was concerned that I could not donate after having had my first chemo and went to do research on it. Happily, when she returned, she showed that we could do it.

To make a long story following a long day short, we made it successfully through the chemo treatment. I followed the advice of all who have gone before and accepted the anti-nausea prescription. It seems to have been a wise decision.

Right now, I don't feel bad at all. I did fall asleep early last night and as a result, was wide awake by 3am. Bruce didn't mind since he got a backrub out of the deal! Still unable to sleep, we sat up and talked, finally getting up about 4:30, and heading out to walk about 5am. We decided that since I am doubly supposed to avoid sun exposure, the early walk would be good for me. It seems to have helped much with the fatigue that I have read and been told comes with chemo.

So far, my only symptoms seem to be a slight nausea, lowered appetite, and increased heart rate. We know that the hair loss is coming in a few days, and have taken the pre-emptive first step to save our plumbing and vacuum cleaner. At 10:30 this morning, using 4 pony tails, my hair was cut off by a professional and set up to be donated. In all, we managed to get

15-16 inches to donate to Locks of Love. She then shaved my head thoroughly and completely amid photo flashes on Bruce's part. We left with me wearing one of the hats that Zoe had selected for the occasion. I have the photos Bruce took to show all who are interested!

The funniest moment of the whole ordeal was when two of the volunteer ladies came around to ask if we would like to have the complementary lunch. I asked Bruce what he thought and when he stated that he didn't know and asked me how much longer I thought it would take, I replied to him, "I don't know because I have never done this before . . ." and then added that he had never heard me say those words before. I wish I had a photo of those ladies' faces too!

26
Random Thoughts on Cancer

So far, the first week after chemo has been surprisingly 'normal'. Yes, I get tired more easily and I do miss my hair, but I have done quite well so far considering the side-effects that I was told to expect.

My body hair has not yet fallen out. If the 'guaranteed' 7-10 days holds true, that should start happening this weekend. (Since I run around at home with my head uncovered, Bruce has reported to me that there is a 'Y' on the top of my head that shows significant thinning.) At least we managed to donate the growth before it fell out so that it will not go to waste. While I have done a couple of rounds with some 'irritable bowels', it has not been anything that I cannot handle, and the medications that were recommended to combat them have worked better than I was told that they would. I am starting to have some very mild mouth irritation, but am drinking my water and sucking on vitamin C like it is candy and seem to be handling it better than they told me to expect.

The one real, continuing problem is that since the chemo started, it is looking more and more like the 'nipple' that the surgeon insisted on 'saving' is not going to make it. I have told the home healthcare nurses that they should expect a call one of these days telling them that my nipple fell off in the shower and asking them what they want me to do with it. Hopefully, when I see the surgeon again next Tuesday, he will have some answers for me.

There are a few areas that my mind keeps going back to while reflecting about the cancer. (I suppose that it is my personal variation on the typical 'why me' that many patients report going through.) I do wonder what I did that upset the trigger and made the cancer show up at all since there is no close family member who has ever had breast cancer. (My grandmother's twin sister had it when she was 86, but the doctors say that she is not closely enough related to count.) The doctors also say that it was present, but dormant for 10-15 years and never showed up until now. If that is true, what was the determining factor that triggered the rapid growth that made it become cancer?

I keep going back in my mind to high school where I was playing in a father-daughter tennis tournament at the Country Club when a very good serve (the ball was probably travelling 100 mph) managed to hit me directly in my left breast. I wonder if that was the beginning of the differences in it. In continued reflecting, it never was as responsive as the other, even when I was breastfeeding my children. (My twisted and warped mind always thought that somehow it realized that the right breast was the family favorite.) I suppose that the different responsiveness may have always been a sign that it was possible that it would develop problems later on. Science hasn't gotten that far in figuring things out from what I can find on the internet to date.

One of the differences in my perspective and other women that I have read about and talked to is how I think about the missing breast. From those I have talked to who have lost a breast to cancer, they consider their breast to have been a vital part of themselves. I look at it more as a closed milk factory that became toxic and needed to be leveled. I really think that having such a perspective is what allows me to keep such a good attitude about the whole thing.

Immediately after my surgery, my surgeon had everyone on high alert to watch me for depression. He had never met someone who could have such an attitude. Knowing that the home healthcare nurses had been told to keep a close watch for depression over losing a breast, along about the third day after I came home, when the nurse was dressing my wound and taking my vitals, I broached the subject with her. I told her that I knew that she had been instructed to watch me for signs of depression. She agreed that she had, so I stated that I supposed that meant that she was reporting back to the doctor about our discussions and my general mood. She agreed that she was. So I told her to report back to the doctor (just to satisfy his need for me to be depressed) that I was terribly depressed. I told her to tell him that I said (in a very flat voice), "Ooooo. Ooooo. I miss my cancer terribly. Can he put it back?"

After reporting back to the doctor, she told me the next day that they no longer were under instructions to watch me for signs of depression.

I have told other friends and confidants that I feel like I am now a life-long member in an exclusive club. I don't remember applying for this membership. The dues are much too steep, and terrible. However, once initiated (even though no one in their right mind would willingly join) you are literally in it for life. Sadly, there is only one way out of this club and that is to join another that is less appealing at this time. Like the song says, "Everybody wanna go to Heaven, but nobody wanna go now."

27
Necrosis Removal

DO NOT READ THIS ONE IF YOU ARE EASILY GROSSED OUT, OR HAVE A WEAK STOMACH!!!

I can still hear the sound of the scissors in the clinic as they snipped away the dead skin from my chest. I knew it needed to be done, but I had no idea that this would be the experience that was nearly my undoing.

Yesterday was pleasant. I taught for the first half of the day and then drove myself to the new surgeon in Odessa to get the information about what to expect with a port going in. One of the first things that she (the doctor) said to me was that she had one year and one month on me (age wise). I liked her immediately and was laughing with her in no time at all! The port will be put in on Friday. Since they want me to report to the hospital between 6:00 and 6:30 am for the outpatient procedure (which should only take about 30 minutes and is scheduled for 8:00 am) I asked my school through an e-mail for volunteers who might be willing to take Zoe in on Thursday night to sleep over, and get her to school the next morning. (Zoe reminded me this morning that her picture day is on Friday.) Two of the lovely ladies with whom I work volunteered to do the deed, and we got Zoe set with a sleepover date. She is very excited that the teacher and her husband have dogs! This will allow Bruce and I to stay in a hotel on Thursday night and get more sleep before reporting to the hospital than would otherwise be possible.

Today was a great day with the students. We are reading novels in each of my classes, and the students are really getting involved in the stories. I missed my last class however because my local surgeon's office called and requested that I come in at 3 pm for my 4:30 appointment since he had a 'procedure' that he needed to do this afternoon. (Little did I know that I was to be that procedure.)

It always feels like I am waiting at one doctor's office or another these days. It has felt that way most of the time since July, when we first discovered the cancer. Today was no exception. I amused myself during the wait by texting with my daughter about the breezy gown that I was wearing, and the temperature of the room; things of that nature. She was laughing at my antics. When it became obvious at about 4:15 that I would not be getting back to the high school any time soon, I called the teacher who was keeping her company and asked her to open my room so that when she got ready to go Zoe would have a 'homey place' to wait for me. At 4:30, the teacher called me back as the doctor walked into the room. I told her that I would call her back and hung up quickly.

Dr. G2 immediately asked how the nipple was doing and I told him that it was not good. I quipped that I was not sure when it was going to fall off in the shower. After climbing back onto the table, he quickly took a look and decided that I was right. It was 'necrotic' and needed to be removed. He told me not to worry about it though, he could do it right there in the office and because the tissues in question were all dead, I would not even need a local anesthetic. What I did need and did not receive were ear plugs and nose plugs. The clever nurses quickly solved one of my issues with the smells by providing me with alcohol wipes to sniff while the work was being done.

The smell was the same bad smell that I have noted when removing the bandages and stepping into the shower. It has been growing worse over the past week or two. It was the smell of rancid meat that you have left in the refrigerator too long before you decide to cook it, or the way that the backyard trashcans get a couple of days after throwing out the packages when you barbecue. The more that he removed, the worse the smell. I went through 2 alcohol wipes; sniffing them against my nose.

Worse than the smell was the sound. Surgeries have never bothered me. Whatever the doctor needs to do is done while I am asleep, so the sounds are never a problem. Being fully awake for this, that was not the situation. Scissors were used. I could tell that they were sharp, but I refused to look as the removal was being accomplished . . . my mind was having a difficult enough time with the awareness of what was happening.

Each sound, each snip, each tug that I felt painted a vivid image in my mind of what was happening to my body. It was at its worst when Dr. G overestimated and hit new tissue with his removal cuts. He was great about backing off of an area when I indicated that he was hitting an area with nerve sensation. He was being very thorough.

Had I known the level of sensory experience I was about to undergo, I would have done two things. I would have taken an anti-nausea tablet, and I would have taken a couple of pain killers…new flesh can be quite sensitive to air exposure. Somehow I managed not to throw-up, although it was pretty high on my list of things to do at some point. I was afraid that if I let it start, the scissors might slip.

There was very little blood involved. The bandaging style has again been changed to no more tape. This time, we used materials that will not fall out each time I turn over or travel to the bathroom. He also ordered a 'wet dressing'. Since the wound has been left open to be sure that there is not additional necrosis, and will not be covered with skin for at least a week, the wet dressing should help to keep the scarring of the under tissues that are now exposed from becoming damaged. I am supposed to return in a week to be stitched up. I am left with bandaging an ugly cylindrical hole where my nipple once was which is now just open tissue that measures about 2 inches in diameter, and is approximately ½ inch deep. Meanwhile, I get to wear a sports bra 24/7 to keep the bandages in place…except for when I shower.

If I can get my mind beyond the smell and the sound, I should be alright.

28
Port in Place (And Other Ramblings)

It has been an interesting week. You already know about the lovely necrosis removal. I received a poster that I had ordered for my classroom and it needs to be trimmed. However, I shudder when I think about using the paper cutter to trim it up nice and even because I think I may pass out when I hear the sound. In my mind, I can just picture the scene. There I am in the teacher workroom and I start to make the first slice . . . the next thing I know, I am surrounded by the administration with the nurse kneeling over me with smelling salts and everyone asking what happened. I would need to refer them to my notes about what I have been through. I don't know if I have the intestinal fortitude to say out loud what the problem is. I think that I will ask around (wimp that I can sometimes be) on Monday and find some other person to trim up the poster when I am not around to hear it!

Today, I had my port installed. In planning for the trip, I had to be sure to wear the right outfit that sends out just the right message. I chose navy capris with a pink shirt with white polka dots so that I could wear a dew rag that was made when I went bald with my friend Vera'. (She lost her battle with metastatic breast cancer in 2007.) The scarf is black with bright, multi-colored polka dot smiley faces. Being somewhat 'folically-challenged' these days, I was allowed to wear my dew rag and a comfy pair of socks into the operating room.

Prior to getting to that point though, we had an interesting start to our day. A wonderful group of colleagues have volunteered to be placed on a standby list of people who are willing to host Zoe overnight should the need again arise. People willing to ensure that she is well fed, well rested, and present at school.

(Within a week of the time we had transferred her to the Fort Stockton schools, Zoe experienced a misunderstanding with a boy she had become friends with. During the misunderstanding, she stabbed him with a pencil. After all of the bragging I had done about what a wonderful, well balanced girl she is, I received a call within a week about her altercation. Fortunately, she had only managed to scratch the boy's arm in the fray. At the time, my boss told her that if she is going to be that aggressive, she needs to be sure that the pencil is very sharp and go for the eyes.)

Even my wonderful boss offered to pencil proof his home and host her! Again, I am feeling overwhelmed at the generosity of the wonderful people with whom I am working!

In addition to the generous list, I received many more gifts this week. My boss's secretary made me the most beautiful blanket that folds into a pillow. (I took that one with me on our trip for the day surgery.) My secret friend gave me another of the wonderful motivational cards with a gift card to Chili's in it! It will help very much to provide a meal for Bruce and me. We decided to use it for lunch after my second chemo next Friday. (All these years and years of battling my weight and watching what I eat and I am now under orders to 'eat it if it sounds good'. Yes. Chemo does come with some blessings!)

Thursday evening, after a quick trip to Sonic, we deposited Zoe with the first of the wonderful volunteers for the night. She was quite happy to be there. Mr. and Mrs. C have two dogs and Zoe was anxious to be walked by them! (She says that she thought that the bigger of the two dogs may have been one that her cousin owned several years ago. She was sure it must be the same dog because, "Their smarts smelled the same!")

Bruce and I had some trouble finding a hotel to stay in. We ended up at the Elegante in Odessa. (Very nice digs.) I told Bruce that he will need to take me back for a romantic weekend after all of this mess is done! Part of the instructions for prepping for the surgery included me showering Thursday evening, and re-showering on Friday morning. This meant that we needed to get up early enough to do the post shower wound care. (Bruce has been doing it a few times per week, so he knew what was needed and we took our supplies with us knowing that we needed to do this.) The problem was that when the hospital called me for the pre-surgical interview, they told me that I needed to be at the hospital and ready surgical prep at 5:30 in the morning. Knowing this, Bruce set the alarm in the room and requested a wakeup call, both for 4:30 am. What we did not notice until I got out of the shower was that the clock in the room was never reset to daylight savings time. So, we were up and showered, and doing our wound care by 4am! (It really sucks to be up and awake that early and not be able to eat or drink!) As requested, the wakeup call came at 4:30am.

We headed to the hospital about 5, and got to wait there some more. (The check in station was not yet open on the surgical floor. There was a kind nurse there who told us where to wait though.) We were only about 10 minutes early for the requested check in. At exactly 5:30 am, we were called back into a room for the pre-op prep.

While most of my healthcare workers have been top notch, the young girl who was assigned to put in my IV for the surgery was more impressed with herself than we were with her. I told her that I have very 'valvy' veins. When she tried to put it into a location that I warned her was not a good place for an IV, she blew the vein and then tried to apply pressure to it with the needle through the vein in an effort to not have to try again. It was very painful, and I have the most terrible bruising on my arm from her arrogance. It will heal with continued use of ice and time.

As I told you, I was allowed to wear my smiley faced dew rag. I told all of my surgical team that it was because I wanted to give them my brightest smiles!

In the surgical prep room (where I spent more time than in the actual surgery) there was another cancer patient. I could not tell for quite a while, because on the way in, Bruce had taken my glasses, so I was flying blind. She had listened to me conversing with the nurse about the cancer, and language, and many other things, and became comfortable enough to begin talking about her own cancer. We struck up a conversation shortly before she was wheeled into her own surgical battle. She was a long time member of the cancer club and told me that hers had not responded as well to the chemo as hoped and that she now has bone metastases. I do not know her name, but please pray for this funny, fantastic lady. Your prayers have helped me so much through all of this and I would like to share!

As they wheeled her close, I could see that she, too, showed a sense of humor and was wearing a turban the size of a shower cap that was silver metallic! It looked as if she was trying to thwart off an alien mind invasion! She also told me about a cancer support group in Midland and invited me to become a part. I explained that I was winging it on my own here in Fort Stockton. She then told me that if I ever get a chance to come out to Midland and play with them, they are calling themselves "The Young and the Breastless". I laughed with her at that one. (It later occurred to me that I only ½ qualify! Wish I had thought to mention that at the time. I think it would have made her laugh!)

When a port is installed, the surgeon keeps you semi-conscious so that you can participate as needed and he or she can gauge reactions to what they are doing. They do give you a mild sedative however that they love to refer to as 'tequila'. When they told me that, I told them that tequila makes my clothes fall off and then looked down at my bare backed, bare butted gown and said, "Oh no...looks like the thought of tequila makes my clothes fall off!"

The strongest nurse in the room is placed in a position of importance. In this case, HE (the only male in the room full of estrogen) was positioned to pull my arm so that it would hold the vein under my clavicle in reach for the doctor. (I asked them if pulling my arm would have the same effect as pulling my finger and they all shouted that they hoped not...said it would be a fire hazard in the OR!) As a result of his good job pulling my arm, I have some small petechial hemorrhages on my thumb. Just means that my thumb ring needs to retire for a week or so.

Long story short . . . well, at least not as long as it could be . . . we were out of the hospital by 11am. We filled my prescription for pain medication at CVS. Dr. G2 was forced to come up with a more reasonable plan for my wound care when we discovered that CVS did not carry the salve that he was wanting me to have for abrading any more potential necrosis...they could order it, but it would not be in until Monday, and would cost us a mere $700.

Speaking of money, Thursday's mail brought us the billing for the first chemo. We don't know what our part to pay will be yet, but the total for that first amount that has been sent to insurance is a mere $3,086.00. (I used to wonder why people with the insurance would have friends and family hold fund raisers to help with bills . . . now I know. This was just 2 office visits and one chemo.) Please add to your prayers one that we win the lottery . . . guess I had better start by buying a ticket!

29
In for a Trim and Cancer Clusters

Another trip to the surgeon.

Last week, I wrote to you about my nipple necrosis. It was not a pleasant experience. Sadly, that seems to be my lot in life for the next little while. Some people make a weekly trip to the barber or hairstylist to get a little trim. I get to go visit the surgeon for a little trim.

Today, I told the doctor that I have finally figured out what the sensation of having the necrotic tissue trimmed is comparable to. If you have ever gone out and ordered a plate of ribs, you know the joy of gnawing on the rib bone after the meat is gone. The sensation of trimming the tissue is comparable to that . . . but from the perspective of the rib bone that is being gnawed. After a short laugh from the doctor when I explained this, he had a much better understanding and was careful to trim much more carefully and quietly.

I have spent a great deal of time in the past week thinking about cancer clusters. Certain communities, certain areas of the State, certain areas of the country seem to have a higher rate and prevalence of cancer. It occurred to me that I have lived my life in the center of a cancer cluster.

The first person I remember knowing who fell victim to breast cancer was a wonderful woman by the name of Ida Mae. Ida Mae was my grandmother's housekeeper. Back in the 60's, women of African American decent were not able to obtain the same level of medical care that everyone now enjoys. Although I was very young when Ida Mae suffered from her untreated breast cancer and subsequently died from it, I remember many of the conversations that took place regarding her situation. She was a very proud lady. She knew that she could never afford the treatments available on her salary as a housekeeper, so she told no one about her condition until it was too late to do anything about it. In her case, the cancer won.

The first true cluster that I recognized was when I was teaching in Shallowater. Three of the four school nurses and our diagnostician all suffered from breast cancer during the same year. It was not all of the same type, but it struck me at the time how hard it had hit our small district. Before the ladies had finished their battles, we had moved to the Austin area and I never knew the outcome of those ladies other than one of them had it metastasize to her liver and had to have ½ of her liver removed.

My next brushes with others suffering with cancer were my first husband and before him, his mother. My ex-father-in-law called my parents to tell them that my ex-husband died from pancreatic cancer. Two of our friends in our Lubbock Sunday School class were admitted to the club. One died of esophageal cancer. Another fought brain cancer. Last I heard, his fight has come back for round two and he lost it last year. (A forth member of the Sunday school class has passed away from colon cancer since I started writing this.) The classroom aide from my Resource room in Shallowater passed away from stomach cancer. Both Bruce's grandfather, and then his father fought the short fight…two months each…with brain cancer. A coworker from the State agency I worked for battled it twice. And then came Vera'.

Vera' was the first person who I joined in her prolonged battle. I regret that I never knew her before she started her fight. I learned so very much from her, and apply her lessons to my current fight. One of the factors that really hit me and continues to haunt my mind is the fact that the FIVE people who used her office in that small school district before her all died from various forms of cancer. (Sounds like an environmental factor to me!) It seems to my mind that clusters can also occur consecutively rather than simply simultaneously.

The cancer club is varied. The one common factor consistently is that the members are primarily wonderful people who have been initiated into the club with no desire to be there. Once admitted though, it is a lifelong membership with very high dues. It is often surprising to meet other members. People in the club often seem to be very private in their fight.

A wonderful woman that I teach with told me today that I need to quit saying that I have cancer. She said that since my margins were clean on the surgery that I need to call myself a 'survivor'. I explained that I am looking forward to doing that once I have made it through the chemo and radiation. She had decided that because I don't show my illness, that I need to think more positively and pronounce myself cured! (I wish it worked that way.)

For right now, I will just keep on keeping on, and occasionally lamenting the fact that where I once had an outie, I now have an innie. If all goes according to the surgeon's report though, today may have been my last trim. If things work out that way, when I go back in next week, I get to look forward to stitches which will turn me from an innie back to flatter than an ironing board. At least when that heals, I should be able to finally get my weighted prosthesis and become a bit less off kilter!

30
Port Support

Today was the official first test drive of the new port for receiving chemo. It took quite a while, but the test was passed . . . finally.

When using the port instead of an IV, the theory is that it is much easier on the patient because there is a ready place to put the IV needle . . . ergo, one stick. As Bruce continued to point out to the struggling nurses (at one time, there were as many as three working on solving the situation), I tend to make things difficult. My one stick turned into a mere five.

The nurses are accustomed to using an older style port that sticks out further than the one that I had received in last week's surgery. The new port is much more streamlined with the center area for needle insertion having large distinctive knobs, and a raised center portion. On the old style, the only soft area is the center where the specialized Huber needle goes. However, when Bard updated its Power Port design, they softened the triangular background and leveled out the top area for greater comfort for the user. It was also placed by my surgeon in such a manner that it will not show under my skin should I choose to wear more 'daring' fashions.

With all of this in my mind, but not known by the nurse, we headed into our chemo session.

Let me back up a minute. We got up early this morning. By early, I mean that I woke up shortly before 4 am and Zoe woke up shortly after I did. One of the stranger seeming symptoms to me is that my left shoulder often hurts at night when I am trying my best to sleep. (One of my nurses explained to me that my surgery was very major and that the muscles that wrap around from front to back were working hard to adjust to the changes in my body.) At any rate, I got up, took a pain pill, and went online for a while; waiting for the medicine to kick in. One of the most comfortable places I have found is my 'spot' in the recliner on the loveseat in the living room. I headed for my most comfortable seat, covered my lap with the wonderful blanket that one of the secretaries at school made for me, and booted up my system. No sooner than I had signed on, I heard Zoe stirring and she appeared at my side saying that she could not sleep. I told her to go lie on the sofa (where she has been stashing her favorite blanket) and she immediately fell into a deep sleep. (In all honesty, I was worried about passing my blood tests . . . tests that I cannot study for, but must pass well in order to be allowed to stay on schedule with my chemo.)

After I, too, fell asleep, Bruce woke to the alarm and came in to wake me up. We allowed Zoe to sleep a bit later than our usual wake up time of 5am. Later, while Zoe put on her school uniform, I selected a purple, grey, khaki, black, and white splash-print shirt, black capris, and my large purple scarf. Bruce was covered in one of his Hurricane Charley tees from the days when he helped restore power to Florida after Charley tried to take out parts of that State, and blue jeans. He ran Zoe by the Donut Palace and on to school on his motorcycle. (She feels like a princess when her daddy drives her to school on the motorcycle!) He then came back to the house to store the motorcycle and get me in the car to make the trip.

Travelling to chemo is like packing for an overnighter. The patient is required to take all medications . . .and there are many . . . something to occupy many an hour, and you can bring a blanket if you choose to. I took the blanket that I used to keep warm while sleeping in my chair. It folds neatly into a pillow, and is oh so warm and soft! I used the time while Bruce was taking Zoe to school to load up the car and clean out some of the week's gathering of trash to make a more comfortable ride. Bruce brought me a delicious and very large breakfast burrito from the Donut Palace run and a bottle of 2% milk. We headed out just before 7:30 for the 95 mile trip to chemo.

We made good time, arriving for the 9:15 appointment at 8:55. When I walked out of the bathroom after checking in, they were already calling my name.

A chemo appointment has 5 components. After checking in, the lab calls you back where they will fill 3 vials with blood and run every blood count known to man. After taking the blood for a test you can't study for, but must pass, you return to the lobby. (Remember, we are toting with us a large bag, purse, and blanket.) About 2 seconds after sitting down and starting to fill out a solid page of possible side effects and marking which ones you have had, you will be called back by a nurse to have the dreaded weight check followed by blood pressure and temperature. (Note to self: Never be telling the story of how the nurse blew your vein last week and told you that it was your problem and not hers while your blood pressure is being taken . . . it will really raise your results!) The nurse escorts you to an exam room where you wait to see the oncologist. This is a good time to compare notes with your chemo partner on what questions need to be asked while having the doctor's undivided attention. The doctor will come in after a short wait and check your test results on his computer and then answer any and all questions. Afterwards, you progress to the fourth component . . . the business manager . . . where you schedule your next appointment and pay for your office visit. (Billing of the chemo will go through the insurance first . . . thank God.) Finally, you will be sent back to the chemo room.

Having passed my test, we were sent to the chemo room where we had been told that the installation of the port was going to simplify and improve the process. Some days, nothing is ever easy with me.

Today's chemo nurse was quite pleased that I now had a chemo port . . . especially since the surgical prep nurse had blown my good veins so badly the week before, rendering them unusable. She explained to me that she would spray a medicine on my skin over my port which would freeze the skin and thus deaden it for the needle insertion. She went on to say that over time, most patients using the port become accustomed to the stick in their chest and no longer need the spray which is good since it can damage the skin when used regularly. This explained, she proceeded to spray, sterilize, stick, and swear . . . she could draw a small amount of blood, but could not clear the line. She was sure that she had inserted the specialized needle properly; however, she removed it and tried again with the same results. Long story short, this process was repeated for a total of four unsuccessful attempts over an hour.

By now, Bruce and I had noticed the nurse who had talked us into having the port installed and raved about how beneficial it would be and how much easier . . . we began to razz her about the fact that it just took her 3 attempts to insert the IV into the vein on the first treatment, but we were about to make attempt number five using the port. I asked her to tell me again how easy, effortless and less painful it was to use the port. Her answer was that since this was just the first time, it would get easier next time.

For the fifth attempt, the nurses decided to try a different process. The section nurse used her left hand to find the outline of two of the sides of the triangular base and while holding it, place the needle in the center of where they had outlined. The first nurse inserted it this way, and the second gave it an additional push in and fastened it down. They had finally inserted it in the proper place. Chemo could begin . . . after they gave me the bag of anti-nausea drugs and steroids. After that, the chemo cocktail was given in two stages . . . the red 'push' drug which a nurse must slowly and manually administer through two large syringes by hand, followed by the second drug which is administered through a bag and IV stand. After all of that, the port must be flushed out and heparin is administered to prevent blood clots from forming in the port's catheter. The entire process takes about 3 hours.

We had some issues with the recliners that are provided for the patients. I am unable to recline it, or stand it back up when I need to get up, so I had Bruce helping me with it. At one point, the chair was so crazy that my feet were over my head and I was at the mercy of Bruce or anyone who might take pity on me and reset the chair.

Later on during the treatment, I had gone to the restroom. My machine liked to beep as soon as I headed to relieve myself...every time. The second time, the machine was saying that it had air in the line. I knew that it would just provide an audible annoyance while I took care of my business, so I did what I needed to do and headed back to my station. My section nurse was doing a push on another patient at the front of our section, and she asked me to stop so that she could fix my machine. I did, and the lady that she was working on commented on my purple scarf. She and her chemo buddy wanted to know where I had gotten it. They thought it was lovely. An older lady sitting across from them piped up her agreement and all wanted to know where I had gotten it and how it worked. I explained to them about Vera' and how I came to make so many different scarfs. I figured that they all see varying stages of hair loss when they take off their own wigs and hats, so I removed my scarf. It is a simple, large square...three feet by three feet...folded into a triangle. I showed them how to position it on the forehead and over the ears and tie it in the back. They asked about materials that they could use and I told them about my smiley face scarf and my pink John Deere. They were delighted and said that they planned to go shop for materials when they finished with their cocktails! I may be a trendsetter for the chemo club!

As a way to play with my progressing male pattern baldness, I have decided to not limit myself. I am adding wigs to the mix. My first has come in. It is blonde and similar to the natural hair that I donated after I started chemo. I plan to also get a red and a brunette in different styles so that I can play and mix things up . . . I do not plan to spend money on Mohawks, or Afros though . . . I might go spikey with one . . . that is wild enough for me!

31
Hair and Meds

Most people have it at some point in their lives. I had it for a while and will get it back again. There was an opera in the 70's by the name. What is it? Hair.

While my oncology doctor has been right about many things, he was off on his timelines. When I started the chemo in September, I was 'guaranteed' that I would lose all of my hair within 7-10 days of the first chemo. Dr. K1 was off on that prediction. I have lost parts and pieces of hair from many different areas of my body. It has simply slowed in some places, and completely fallen out in others, but I am not yet hairless.

There are many aspects of the hair loss that are simply not discussed. Vera' had filled me in about a few, so I had a better idea of what to expect than most people do. For example, pending hair loss is known to the patient when they start to lose their most private area hair.

I have known for some time that I suffer (or rather everyone around me suffers) from my overdeveloped sense of humor. It has recently come to my notice that I also have a rather overactive imagination.

When the discomfort of the pending hair loss in my most private areas made itself known, I began to have rather overactive imaginings of potential scenarios in my head that, thankfully, did not come to be. To prevent them, I would daily wear my most accommodating granny panties to ensure that they would not come to pass. You see, I was living a walking dread-dream that I would be leaving little bunnies of the hair behind me as I walked down the halls of the school, and I really didn't want to leave the physical evidence, much less need to explain to anyone what was going on! In this case, a pound of good underwear was worth an ounce of prevention

. . . or something like that!

I have not needed to shave my underarms for a few weeks now. That is one area where I was glad to see the hair go. That and my legs, and my old lady mustache and beard! No plucking, no waxing, equals much time saved in the shower. I have lost my right eyelashes, but still have my left, and both eyebrows. The top of my head is stubbly in places and smooth as a baby's bottom in others. As time has gone on, I am much less self-conscious about it than I was in the beginning. I may even spend a day or two as the totally bald woman in school before it is all said and done. Let's face it, wigs are scratchy and scarves and hats can get too hot. One of the wonderful teachers in my department commented yesterday when I was having one of my take the scarf off moments that she doesn't understand why I don't just 'rock-it' with the shiny bald head. I may do that once the rest of the hair falls out…right now, it is still too patchy for my taste.

Last week, I learned a very important lesson. I had been sneezing and sneezing. I was becoming concerned that I might be getting a cold. (At chemo, you are instructed to contact the oncology offices about ANY signs of an illness. Never assume that it is allergies. Always call them to get their take on it . . . I am not very good at following that advice so far, but did finally do that today . . . but I will tell you about that in a minute.) Anyway, I was sneezing and sneezing. My nose itched something fierce. I was glad that I didn't call the doctor's office though when I finally figured out that I was losing the hairs in my nose . . . it was an itchy process!

On another subject, I have found another one of those medical issues that everyone forgets to mention. It seems that because I had the port installed, my oncologist decided that I needed to be on blood thinners. After following the prescription since last Friday, I called them this morning and told them to come up with another plan.

Not everyone can take blood thinners safely. It seems that in my case, my body responds with racing heart and soaring blood pressure. When my home health nurse told me yesterday afternoon after my hot shower and down time while waiting for her that my blood pressure was 158/88 and that I might need to stay home for a few days, I knew that it was time to call the oncologist's office. During 3rd period, our inclusion aide covered the classroom while I went to have my BP checked. I was down to 155/77. Having talked to the nurse at Dr. K1's offices, I did not take the Coumadin today (at lunch is when I have been taking it), and by the time I went to the surgeon's office, my blood pressure was 117/72. (If it should have been up at any time, it should have been up then . . . I had another trim today!)

On a more positive note, Dr. G2 said that all of the necrosis was gone with today's trim. He has left the decision of whether or not to stitch up the healing wound to me. With stitches, he said that I should only need bandages for another 3 weeks. Allowing it to heal on its own, I will be in bandages for at least another 6 weeks. Looks like next Tuesday, I am getting stitches.

32
I Made the Centerfold!

It has been another crazy week here. Now we are at the weekend that starts my favorite week . . . the week before my next chemo. This is the week when I feel more like myself again. I still get tired easily, but I think that at least part of that is due to the off balance issues that I mentioned earlier. Another part is that my body is doing its best to play catch up and send things back to normal in my system.

I have had enough people telling me that I am not handling chemo like a 'normal' person that I am starting to believe them. It should have never been in question though, since no one has ever accused me of being normal! The counselors at school, upon finding out that I have daily home healthcare, asked me if my nurse was a young, good-looking man. When I told them no, and asked why they thought that, they told me that they were looking for the reasons that I am doing so very well with the chemo and not missing work, terribly sick, and other 'normal' responses to the chemo. I laughed with them and told them that I am still just on the first chemo cocktail. It may be the one that I switch to after Thanksgiving that does me in. Time alone will tell.

One of the best things about being on the chemo is that for the first time in my life, I am under doctor's orders to 'eat it if it sounds good'. The flip side of that is that there is not a whole lot that sounds good. I don't have much appetite, but I have found that by eating good proteins several times a day, I am able to rebuild my blood supply and maintain a fairly normal lifestyle. I still go walking on the track on the weekends with Bruce, I have not missed any time from work so far other than the days that I go and get my chemo.

My hair loss is still spotty . . . in other words, all of the gray hair fell out, and my stubble thinned, but it didn't all fall out . . . at least not yet. I did have an interesting wake up the other night. I rolled over and flopped my arm on my pillow and wound up with a face full of fallen out fluff from the back of my head. Made me sputter and cough, and then I had a laughing fit. It reminded me of something from an old Carol Burnett skit. In fact, the biggest problem that I have had over the past week is waking up at night with one funny thought or another in my head. It is an interesting experience when you wake up laughing in the middle of the night!

The growth of the remaining hair has slowed down. (I still use the electric razor on my legs once a month or so.) However, while thinner, I still have some hair in all of the normal hair places. I content myself with the knowledge that at least I no longer need to pluck or wax my face!

Another bonus for the face . . . for the whole body for that matter . . . is that chemo is like having a total body chemical peel. I did shed some skin for a while (nothing major), and now my skin is better than I remember it ever having been before! I don't know what the recommended lotion will be when I have the radiation (I understand that it causes some burns that need special treatment with certain lotions), but for the time being, I love using Gold Bond Ultimate healing. It smells like roses, and it feels wonderful. (I even use it on my bald head for a special skin treat!)

The most prevalent symptom of being on chemo is that I get really tired each day and find myself going to bed earlier and earlier each night. I start out the week going to bed around 10, and end the week falling asleep around 8:30. (Part of that may be due to the waking up laughing in the middle of the night a couple of nights per week . . . who knows?)

This week, I received the honor of having an article written about me by a former student and placed in the school's newspaper, The Tumbleweed. (Pretty good name for a school newspaper in a desert town!) After receiving a copy, I told my bosses that I am so honored and surprised. I am sure that my parents will be proud to know that I finally made the 'centerfold' in a printed publication. (Yes, Mom, I got an extra copy for you and Dad!) It was very nicely written, and I am proud of the young lady who wrote the story. She did a very nice job and made me sound pretty good! (Now, if only she were passing her current English class I would be a happy former teacher of hers!)

While we are making trips to get the chemo, my innie has finally been sewed up, and I am in 'surprisingly good shape' all things considered, I am starting to feel that old feeling of being in a holding pattern again. I spend a bit of time wondering if the chemo is doing what it is supposed to do, and if we are winning this war. I do wish that there was some magic way to know what the status of my cells is as we are going through this process. For now, I just need to be satisfied that I am feeling healthy, still have my sense of humor, and that God is taking care of the rest. (I know that everything is going to turn out the way it is supposed to . . . I just wish that I had more control of what all is going on!)

Maybe that is the lesson in all of this for me . . . that I tend to have some control issues and that I need to better learn how to let go and let God. I don't really know. What I do know is that I have seen many positive things come from this diagnosis. Maybe the lesson is in looking for the positive when the situation looks so negative. All I know for certain is that I am very blessed and very grateful for all of the blessings that I have been given and continue to receive! I am a very lucky lady!

33
The Stitches

It occurs to me that while I told you that I have had my 'innie' stitched up to flat-board status; I never told you how that process worked out.

I had decided upon going in to have the stitches that I would make sure that I did not end up with any further phobias (such as my fear of the sound of scissors), so I took my mp3 player with me. I did not, however, get it out. I had been worried about what I might hear, and what sensations I might experience. I did not need to waste so much energy on the worry, however.

Dr. G2, even though the extent of feeling in my surgically altered side is not sure at this point, gave me local anesthetic. Thankfully, what feeling is there is too uncertain to be something that I can specify yet. I did feel something of a cold burn when the medicine went in. It was not bad . . . I would not want to experience it again . . . but it was not too terrible.

After being numbed-up, I decided that what I had needed with the necrosis and did not request was prayer. With that in mind, as they began to prep me for the stitches, I closed my eyes and placed myself in a semi state of self-hypnosis from which to pray. I closed off the sounds and most of the sensations and invited God to hold my hand . . . to hold me and take away my fears and trepidations over the procedures. (I also apologized for not inviting Him to comfort me sooner and reminded him of my stubborn streak!) A great, wonderful calm descended over me, and then a very strange thing began to happen.

As I laid there and prayed, calming myself, Dr. G2 began to speak. He told me a story of a lady who had come to him several years ago with very serious problems. He said that all of the tests showed a life-threatening situation that required quick and decisive surgical action. After showing her the test results and going over them with her, she promised to come in the next day for surgery, but told him that she needed to take the night to pray and commune with God.

He continued his story speaking to me in low, soothing tones. He told me that the woman reported for her surgery the next morning. Using the CAT scan results, and x-rays to pin point the numerous areas of concern, he proceeded with the surgery. Upon opening her body up and going in to operate, all of the numerous bad places were gone. He said that they searched and searched, but were unable to find any problems in any of the places where the tests showed her illnesses. Additional scans and tests showed no sign of her previous problems.

Dr. G2 continued, saying that he went to visit the woman and ask her if she knew why she was so ill one day and had no evidence of the illness the next. She simply told him that she supposed that it was God's will.

The thing that struck me most as Dr. G2 stitched and spoke, as I had been praying, was the topic of the story that he chose to tell me as I was lying there and quietly saying my own prayer. I do not believe in coincidence. Instead, I believe that I was receiving an answer to my request for comfort and calm.

The process of getting the stitches was a calm and rather comforting experience. In addition to the unusual conversation, I now have the comfort of knowing that the days of bandages are numbered. Today marks 72 days that I have lived with the bandages. I have watched them grow smaller, yet I have scars from the tape that holds them on. They have been a double edged sword in this long, drawn-out healing process. Tomorrow, and day 73, marks another trip to the surgeon. Maybe he will remove the stitches . . . maybe not, but I am comforted by knowing that the days of healing still to go from my mastectomy are numbered.

34
Questions Answered

Today marked the third round of chemo cocktail number one. That leaves only one more round of the Adriamycin and Cyclophosphamide, and then chemo cocktail one is done. The final round will be on November 4 . . . a day that has always been important to me, but will now take on an additional significance. After that, we will start chemo cocktail number two with a different schedule.

Overall, for a chemo day, Bruce and I are feeling great and highly optimistic! We took a list of questions to ask Dr. K1 and the answers we finally received were better than we hoped.

We arrived early at the Cancer Center, and checked in. After paying, we were able to get coffee, go to the restroom, and just start filling out the required paperwork listing a full page's worth of possible (to be expected in most people) side effects common to many people who receive chemo. (It is a rather intimidating list that must be completed every visit so that the oncologist can more accurately monitor your progress and reactions to the chemicals you are receiving. Thankfully, mine usually has very little marked!) I was then called back for my prerequisite test. Three blood vials later, I rejoined Bruce in the main lobby.

We did not have a very long wait until we were called back to the not so fun process of the dreaded 'weigh-in' followed by vitals. As we sat through those, the nurse told us about an earlier patient who decided to balk at having a blood pressure check. (At the time we took it as small talk rather than a heads-up about some serious wait time!) After the vitals, we were taken to an exam room to meet with Dr. K1. (He's better at grading than I am . . . results of the tests are usually within an hour . . . of course the computer does it for him.)

Today was a different matter. I sat. I paced. I read over our list of questions. I read a magazine article about how the brain works in optimistic people while leaning on the counter and exercising my legs. I left and went to the rest room. I came back and checked status updates on Facebook while leaning on the exam bed and exercising my legs. I read e-mail. Etc...etc...etc. Bruce showed tremendous patience and sat perfectly still while reading a financial magazine. Finally, one and one-half hours after we checked in, Dr. K1 made it into the room.

Dr. K1 is a soft-spoken, smallish man. He walked into the room apologizing profusely and stating that we had the misfortune of coming in directly behind TWO sets of patients who decided to be 'difficult'. I immediately looked at Bruce and said, "See, I told you, Honey, that I need to find ways to be more difficult to get better service!"

Dr. K1 almost shouted out, "NO!!! No, no, no, no! Please don't do that! Not only will you not get better service, but we will be saying bad things about you after you leave!"

After we laughed a minute, and chatted some more while Dr. K1 was accessing the computer results of my morning's tests, we got down to the business at hand. (By now, I must tell you that I was VERY proud of Bruce . . . he does not normally wait very patiently, but he was good as gold!) To sum up our list of questions, we asked about which of the two most prevalent medications would be the next cocktail, and I had some concerns about results from the initial testing and where I stand with the cancer.

The two taxanes that are usually used for the second chemo cocktail are derived from the pine tree, or the yew tree. I am constantly confusing their names, and since I was writing the list of questions as we were driving to Odessa, I was not where I could Google the correct name, so I simply asked him whether we were looking at using pine or yew. He told us that he prefers pine (it has milder side effects for most patients) but that he had recently read that there might be a shortage of pine in the US this year. If that turned out to be the case, then we would use the yew, but only if the pine were not accessible. So the preferred chemo for round two will be

Taxol. (Now you can look it up and see all of the fun side effects that I will need to watch for and possibly experience during round two if you are interested!)

Another of our primary questions came from some concerns that I have not really gone into with you up to this point. Back in July, before the mastectomy, I had begun to experience a numb spot on my chest. Prior to the surgery, I mentioned this numbness (which feels something like I had received a shot of Novocain to the area) to Dr. G2. He, of course, told me not to worry about it. Evidently he did the worrying for me. When the surgery was done, he traced a "thread" from one of the affected lymph nodes into the muscle wall where I had indicated the numbness to him. He removed the thread and surrounding tissue and the area in the muscle wall that I had indicated. It was concerns over this and the indication that I had received from Dr. P and Dr. G2 that there was a possible bone involvement in my sternum. I wanted answers and I wanted the bottom line . . . so, when I felt that I was finally ready to hear the answers, I asked. That was today.

Translating medical reports almost requires an advanced degree, and Dr. K1 was happy to set the record straight. He even printed out a copy of the report for us.

The 'scary places' on my bone scan around my sternum were actually marks on one of my ribs that the medical team felt were due to an old and possibly forgotten or ignored injury. Bruce immediately leapt to remembering another weird medical condition that I have battled where I would not reabsorb shed bone cells like a normal body does. (After my wonderful sister-in-law spent hours upon hours researching the condition, I began to take large quantities of vitamin B (sublingual) and managed to clear up that old complaint.) Bottom line was that there was no evidence of a bone metastasis.

The 'thread' that went into the muscle wall was so microscopic that the margins from the surgery were completely clean, and there was no evidence of it on the CAT scan. In other words, He told me that unless and until he tells me otherwise after I have completed all of my chemo and radiation and have had additional scans that show otherwise, I am to consider myself and call myself a cancer survivor. I have survived Stage III breast cancer. I am undergoing the chemo and the radiation to prevent a recurrence and remove any other microscopic shoots that may have found their way into my system before the surgery . . . but I am to consider myself a breast cancer survivor! (Those words feel like a song, a poem, a prayer, a gift, a miracle from God!)

I guess that the teacher at school who told me to quit saying that I have cancer and start calling myself a survivor was right!

35
Chemo Three

After the third round of chemo, we have come to the conclusion that we will never be able to plan any other activities to do while we are in Odessa on chemo days. It seems that what should take about two hours for most people . . . three at the most . . . will always take the majority of the day for me. My appointments are always scheduled for 9-9:30 am. We have yet to be able to leave before 2 pm, so we give up. Our chemo days will henceforth be dedicated to chemo and nothing else.

While the first round using the port took five attempts to access, this time it only took two. We now know that in order to access my port, I need to be lying in the chair with my feet over my head and the nurse holding two sides of the triangle of the port while accessing the center. (It is a bit like practicing contortionism.)

B was my nurse of the day. We spent a long time just waiting to get started. (I told you last time how Dr. K1 was dealing with two sets of difficult patients before us.) It was nearly 11:30 before we were finally in the chemo room and B was attempting to access my port. For a 9:15 appointment, that seemed rather excessive to us. (I was so very proud of Bruce. He does not have a large amount of patience, and he bore the delays in stoic silence.)

After my port was accessed, we had a 20 minute wait while I was administered my IV of anti-nausea drugs and steroids. Once that was done,

B changed things up and gave me what I have until this point had last first, saving the push on the Adriamycin for last. While I was receiving my IV, the volunteers came through and brought sandwiches to us all. Bruce and I both chose to have peanut butter and jelly.

We had some issues this session with the Adriamycin push. As the nurse started the push, thankfully, she noticed the drip from the syringe onto the sleeve of my shirt and the arm of the chair. Also thankfully, it did not drip on me. (Saved by my sleeve!)

Adriamycin is such a tough chemical that it is the reason that I needed to get the port installed. Any contact with skin can cause chemical burns that can lead to permanent nerve damage, extreme scaring, and all kinds of other unpleasantness. It is bad enough that it instantly stained the arm of the chair, and as she cleaned it up off of the chair and my sleeve, B was required to change her gloves 3 times. (She was told that it could absorb through one set of gloves in only a couple of minutes.)

In trying to establish the cause of the leak, the first guess was that it was the connection on the side of the tubing. The process was stopped while the tubing connecting to my port was changed and a different access was made available. Another nurse that B reported to, who also advised her about changing her gloves, provided the plastic bottomed spill protection sheets to cover my arm as we resumed the push. The arm of the chair had a new, probably permanent stain, and I was given instructions on how to wash my shirt . . . twice and by itself. (And they are injecting this directly into my system!)

Changing the tubing did not solve the problem of the leak. Since double gloving was called for for B, she added an extra sheet over my arm to help protect me. It was determined that when the syringe was loaded, the pharmacy tech who loaded it must have broken the outermost tip off of it which caused the drip. There was not any problem with the push of the second syringe.

Our next problem happened after the port had been cleaned and the heparin had been administered to prevent clots in the port. B removed the special needle from the port. There was a backwash from my veins. B had never experienced this before and had assumed that since it was a port, it would not bleed when the needle was removed. She removed the needle with nothing handy to stop any blood flow.

Having just received the chemo, my blood was as toxic to the rest of humanity as the actual chemicals that had just been administered to me. Things were flowing pretty good. I managed to pick up my bra strap just getting the edge soaked in the blood. The remaining pool sat on my skin over my port until B was able to grab some gauze from a cart and clean it up. In all, it may have taken all of a minute to a minute and a half to clean up the mess and stop the flow with a Band-Aid.

We all had a laugh about how some people just seem to attract trouble. This time, that person seems to be me. Bruce wasted no time in teasing me by telling everyone that I tend to be one of those people who just causes issues from time to time . . . or in my case, every three weeks. We wrapped things up, gathered things up and headed out.

It is interesting to note that the first couple of days after chemo are not too bad. In all honesty, since I take my chemo on Friday, the following Monday is usually the hardest day for me. Bruce and I get up and go walking on Saturday morning, and Sunday morning, but Mondays seem to kick my bootie. This round was no exception.

One thing that was different this time though was that by Tuesday, the skin over my port itched so badly that I could have chewed nails. Thoughts of clawing the skin were jumping through my mind. I did not know what I could possibly do, so I called the oncology offices and asked to speak to Dr. K1's nurse.

As with any call to any doctor's office, I left a voice mail and decided that my itch was so severe that I would even take the call back during class if I had to (something that I will normally not do unless it is an emergency because I don't think that it would be right for me to be taking phone calls when the students are not allowed to.) This time, however, I considered the situation to be an emergency!

True to Murphy's Law, the nurse called me back at the beginning of a class. Fortunately, it was one in which I have an inclusion aide with me. I apologized to the class and headed out to the hall to take the call.

In discussing the situation with the nurse, I was glad that I had called. It turns out that I was dealing with a potentially dangerous situation from the seepage onto my skin and was having a reaction to the chemo on my skin. I was told to get Benadryl Cream and some Hydrocortisone and blend them under a bandage. Also, I needed to monitor the site for redness, heat, or peeling. After just 48 hours of this treatment, things were back to a more normal state of repair.

Yesterday, Pecos County Medical Hospital had their first annual "Get up and Walk, Run, or Stroll" in the park. Bruce had to work, but Zoe and I headed to the park and participated in the Three Mile. Events included a One Mile, a Three Mile, and a Five Mile. In all, there were 48 registered participants. Zoe came in 25th, and I came in a bit behind her with another breast cancer chemo patient from San Antonio at 29th. The completion medals are beautiful, and Zoe won $25.00 as the first girl to complete in her age group. I feel like I won as well. My pedometer indicated that the 3 mile track was actually 4.96 miles . . . but my partner and I did get lost at one point and probably added a bit to our mileage. (We were not the only ones who managed to lose the trail. At one point, I know I saw one of the Five mile runners pass a certain area twice!)

I am really looking forward to the 'feeling better' week this week, and the 'feeling best' week next week before my round four of chemo cocktail number one. I'll keep you posted.

36
Back in Balance

I finally have a prosthesis! Growing up, I never imagined that I could get so excited at having matching boobies at the age of 48. Who knew?!

This morning, we headed out at our usual time to make eye exam appointments for Zoe and me in Odessa at 9 am. It was time for our annual exam. Zoe had been in the primping-pre-teen-beautifying stage and wanted to get contacts again to go with her new haircut and tendency to spend excessive amounts of time in front of mirrors trying to look her best. It was simply time for my annual eye exam.

Zoe's eye prescription needed to be tweaked a bit. (Being nearsighted tends to do that to a person annually.) For the first time in as long as I can remember, mine did not need to be changed at all! (Whoot!) I get to spend another year at the same strength. Dr. A was also pleased with the overall checkup because he said that often, chemo tends to cause the tear production to dry up, but mine is going fine. (He also commented that while this is unusual, just praise God and keep on trucking!)

Part of the beauty of using an eye doctor in a mall is the ability to make Saturday appointments. With all of the delays we have experienced each time we have gone into 'town' for a chemo treatment, we have learned not to try and accomplish anything else while we are there. There simply isn't time after chemo. We always need to rush home so that we can be here in time to pick up Zoe from school. (I am sure that we could probably find someone here to watch her until we get home, but we are saving our requests for some time when we may really need to ask for help. I have a list of people who have volunteered that was developed when Bruce and I needed to spend the night in Odessa before my port was put in.)

We managed to finish with both eye exams before 10 am, so we walked to the store where I would be fitted for my new prosthesis and arrived before they were open. As I sat to wait for them, Bruce and Zoe headed off to find where Radio Shack was so that I would not get overly tired because of walking around trying to locate the places we needed to go.

I did not have a long wait.

Buying a new limb was a new experience for me. Having never before required one, I was not certain how the process works. My caseworker at the American Cancer Society has been wonderful, and talked me through much of the preliminaries of the process. I found it strange and amusing that I was required to obtain a prescription from one of my doctors in order to purchase a prosthetic breast! But, that was one of the wonderful things that I learned about this process. The best part is that by having the prescription and filling out the paperwork in advance (we faxed back and forth several times), the American Cancer Society will provide me with a prosthesis every 3 years, and two new mastectomy bras each year. (The prosthesis runs from about $150 for a basic breast, up to around $400 for a custom made. It just depends on what you want, what you need, and what you can afford.) If I am able to find a place to swim, I will need to purchase a 'swim prosthesis' which is made from a different material and can only be used in chlorinated water. If we decided to take a trip to the coast, I will need to plan ahead and order one that can be used in salt water. I have been told that the only place to find those is to order from England. (At this point in time, it looks like we will need to add a suitcase to our travels . . . one for our clothes and toiletries, and another for two to three spare breasts. This lends a whole new meaning to 'save the ta-tas'!) Prosthetic breasts must be kept in their box at night to help retain their shape, and unless they are designed for swimming, they must not get wet.

Another lesson for the day was that mastectomy bras do not fit like other bras. They do require a fitting . . . but then so do new boobies. By the time we found and settled on the first bra and prosthesis, Bruce and Zoe were back. The lovely lady who was doing my fitting had me put my shirt back on and then go model for Bruce. (Her reasoning was that no one on earth can judge a good prosthetic breast fit like a husband!) Believe it or not, Bruce judged the first one to be too large. Something about the shape was just not right.

The owner of the store is in the process of selling her inventory and there was not a prosthesis available in the next size down. To try and work around this problem without having to special order and wait two more weeks (remember, I have been 'without' since August 1 and was rather anxious to finally have something more substantial than stuffing in my bra), we found another prosthetic breast in the same size, but a different brand. This new one was somewhat heavier than the first, but has a wrap-around quality that fills in the hole that was left under my arm. We loaded it into the new bra and after putting my shirt back on again; headed back to the front for Bruce's input. He was nodding his head as I walked through the door. We found a match! After more paperwork, and visiting a bit with the clerk, we were off and I was less off kilter than I have been in quite awhile.

Knowing that we were going in for a fitting today, and hoping to be successful, rather than wear one of the wigs, I travelled in a scarf. As we headed into the fitting process I just described (the clerk and I), when I removed my scarf to try on boobies and bras, she commented on my fuzzy head. Even though I have one more round of the A-C, and still have all of my T to go, I am getting fuzzy headed again. (This time on the outside rather than brain-wise . . . although I still have a certain amount of that too!) After looking closely, the clerk pronounced it to be light red. When she stated this to Bruce, he simply told her that it would fit my personality since I tend to have a 'red-headed temperament'. To quote a very wise woman (Forrest Gump's mother), "Life is like a box of chocolates. You never know what you gonna get."

37
Chemo Cocktail One is Done

Is it considered politically correct to say 'hurrah' and 'yuck' in the same breath?

Today was the final round of the Adriamycin. As I found out shortly after the push (I had only suspected before), this particular chemo builds up in your system to nasty levels. That is why treatments are each three weeks apart, and why it takes a bit more time for bounce back each time a new treatment is administered. This time, I really felt it!

The Adriamycin had been pushed into my system and I was receiving the Cytoxan when full blown nausea hit me. I managed to keep it all in, but wondered (as I often do) what things looked like from Bruce's perspective . . . watching me all pink cheeked when we got there and growing paler by the minute. I knew it was fairly dramatic this time when I went to the restroom the last time and looked in the mirror as I washed my hands . . . wow. Like a ghost. Wearing my blonde wig looked good with my coloring when we got there, but not so much anymore. (It was rather creepy in an 'Adams Family' sort of way . . . keeping the theme with my new 'Cousin It'.)

For those of you who don't know, after 82 days in bandages, I finally managed to get my new prosthesis last weekend. It is a lovely shade of pale pink, weighs four pounds (I have weighed it repeatedly), and moves much more like a real breast than the stuffing that I used before. As part of the celebration, I held a fun 'name that prosthesis' contest. There were many interesting, funny and enthusiastic suggestions made. Some were very good, indeed. The best suggestions were the following: Mabel, Side Saddle Annie, Harmony, The Imposter, Thing One and Thing Two (even though there could only be a Thing One at this point in time), Edna, Maxine, Jamie's Jug, Betty Boob, Twin Sister, The Other, Pinkie, and Bruce's Little

Buddy among others. The winner though was from here at home. Zoe's winning suggestion came from her love of the "Adams Family" movies. My prosthesis is now called "Cousin It". (One hilarious post from a dear OLD friend from high school who posted the following query: "Will you start keeping the "original" in a box now that you know this helps retain shape?")

On days like today when I am feeling on the 'yuck' side of life, I get a huge pick-me-up from going back and reading all of the fun and funny things that my friends have had to say about this ordeal . . . sort of like a roast for the dearly, clearly departed who has been replaced by 'Cousin It'. I believe that the main reason that I have done so well on chemo is that I have not lost my sense of humor!

A great deal of credit for the lack of side-effects goes also to my students. For many people, work is what you do when you can't be home. I love home as much as the next person, but to me the quickest path to feeling sorry for myself and wallowing in a self-pity pot would be to have to stay home and feel bad there. My students keep me going. Some days it is hard to get up, but I remind myself that those kids need me and deserve the best I can give them and that challenge helps me to pull the best out for them. (I readily admit that my 'best' this year seems to have physical limitations that I am learning to work around, but I still need to give them the best that I can. They deserve no less!) No matter how lousy I am feeling when I get up, I have one student first period who always greets me with a huge smile and laugh about whatever wig I have worn, or scarf, or turban. It always gets the day off to a good start.

My next chemo will be on December 2. I will have one each Friday for 3 weeks, with one week off at Christmas. Then I will start it up again the following week. This will happen in this pattern for four times. If all goes according to plan and I am able to keep to the schedule, I should be starting radiation during Spring Break. The counseling department at school will be happy to know that (again, if I can keep to schedule) I should complete my radiation the week before the new state assessments in April.

We have made it through steps one and two. Now we just have steps three and four . . . we are half-way! Thank you for all of your love, prayers, and support. I don't know if we could be doing it without you!

38
Fingertips and Neuropathy

A couple of the more interesting points in dealing with all of the cancer treatments are the continuing neuropathy from the mastectomy and the changes in my fingertips from the chemo.

I find that these days I spend a great deal of time looking at my fingertips. It has been a gradual change, but as promised, the chemo has changed them: bits and pieces at a time.

The first change is in the quality of the nails. There is none left. My nails are brittle and heavily lined. I find myself fascinated by the purplish shade of the growth crescents at the base of the nails . . . these were once a nice shade of peachy-white. The nails themselves have more curve to them than they have ever had before. I have managed to keep them long so far, but it is not looking too good for the home team right now. They are starting to crack low, below the quick line. I suspect that they will need to be cut down soon to prevent the coming breakages from doing serious damage.

The other side of my fingertips has darkened too. The home health nurses say that this is a normal part of the chemo process and that it should reverse after the process is over and my body begins to heal again. Most fascinating to me is the wrinkles that have developed across the tips. These wrinkles remind me of the ones that I used to get from spending too much time in the swimming pool. I wonder if it will change my finger prints. Occasionally, I will get red spots (similar to red bruises) which show up on my fingertips.

The other thing that gets my undivided attention is the neuropathy from my surgery.

Whenever a doctor removes something as large as a breast, he must work hard to not damage the main nerve that runs through it, nor the main blood vessel that runs through. These are, as my surgeon described, two of the biggest challenges faced during the surgery by the surgical team. Because many, many, many small nerves (the branches if you will) are removed with the breast tissue, it takes an exceedingly long time for normal sensations to be felt in the area of the surgery. Much of the information says that many patients never recover 'normal' sensation again.

In the case of my surgery, I have developed some interesting sensations to go with my interesting scars. There are places where you can touch my back and it feels numb to me . . . as if I have just been given Novocain in that spot. I have one area that we discovered with my wound treatment on the side, toward the front, where it feels as if you were rubbing my shoulder blade in back. These first began to show around the time that my drainage tubes were removed. But there is one place that I am not sure how to act when it is touched. You see, I was never ticklish before, but I am ticklish now.

It is quite startling to suddenly become ticklish at the age of 48 when you were never ticklish before. It can sneak up on you. For example, when in the shower soaping up and the bar runs across the new tickle spot under your arm and you find yourself squealing like a young girl because you have just managed to tickle yourself. (The giggles are not nearly as embarrassing as the flinging of the bar of soap across the shower and then trying to not injure yourself as you collect it from the floor!)

When wearing 'Cousin It', or my exercise prosthesis, the tickle spot does not bother me. It is better protected from accidental contact under the thick layers of silicone that serve to give the appearance of having a breast. (This makes me think that I may have always been ticklish, but had thick enough layers of fat covering me that they were impenetrable and thus, impervious to the sensation of being tickled.)

Most of the time, this is just a silly inconvenience. On one occasion, however, it became quite an amusement to me and two of my home health nurses.

Back when I was still being bandaged, shortly after the innie had been sewn shut, we had an 'incident' one evening when the home health nurse had come to change the dressing. Because of the extensive time in tape, I was having issues with my skin dissolving underneath the tape and we had gone through a variety of fixes. A new solution had been invented by the nurses and was working well, but we did not have enough materials to do the job properly, so my nurse of the evening called for another nurse to bring over the items we needed to complete the bandage. We became heavily involved in telling stories and cracking jokes while we were waiting, and we continued after the other nurse arrived. (We were having such fun that the second nurse stayed to play the word games and swap stories with us while we took care of my bandages.)

As the nurse was finishing with my bandages and applying the tape, she was engaged in telling a funny story. The second nurse was standing by and laughing as my nurse began to punctuate her point. What she did not realize was that she was punctuating with her finger on the bandage which was right over my ticklish spot. I began laughing, thrashing, and kicking my foot up in the air. (I was raised that it is rude to interrupt, so I simply kicked helplessly and laughed and thrashed and prayed that her story would end so that I could breathe again!) The second nurse stood by laughing almost to the point of hysterics. She could see what was going on, but evidently she, too, had been raised to not interrupt. She, too, was laughing helplessly. After what seemed like forever, the story finally ended. As it ended, the punctuation on the bandages ended too. (Finally, oxygen to my lungs!)

Once the story ended, the second nurse (amid much giggling), told the first nurse what was really happening as she told her story. She was very embarrassed about it, and remains so to this day (although I tell her to embrace the humor of the situation!)

That's enough about me. For now, life in the real world beckons. I have a lovely preteen who needs to get a bra that fits . . . and doesn't have underwire. (I still believe that underwire adds to the factors that create growth opportunities for breast cancer.)

39

Canceritis

One of the more common issues during recovery from a cancer diagnosis is "Canceritis". This is the belief that any new lump, bump, sniffle, or sneeze is the cancer coming back up in another place, or another form. Let's face it . . . cancer is scary!

Tuesday morning, I found myself suffering from a very strong case of Canceritis.

Day before yesterday, in an effort to fight back against the weight gain that comes with the chemo, my daughter and I began going to the high school pool for some after-hours swimming. It was rather amazing to see all of the people who were there. One of the best discoveries was the water aerobics class that was going on. I joined in and had a wonderful workout!

After returning home and getting into the shower to rinse off the chlorine (can't have my new fuzzies turning green), I discovered a painful lump under my right arm. (This would not have been such a scary thing were it not for the fact that my cancer was all on my left side.) Painful; not good. Lump in armpit; not good. Painful lump in armpit while in between chemo treatments; REALLY not good!

Because it was night, I waited until the next morning to call a doctor. Part of the problem was deciding on which doctor to call. I finally settled for calling my oncologist's office. I called just before 8am and left a message with the answering service, and tried not to freak-out too badly while I waited for the nurse to return my call.

So far, I think that I have handled this cancer business with a fairly level head. I have managed to continue working; only taking off on the days that I have received my chemo and the day I got my port installed. Otherwise, I have been fortunate to remain rather functional compared to other chemo patients that I have talked to, read about, and known. I try to keep an analytical perspective of the process with an eye toward the ridiculous and/or amusing aspects of treatments. However, from the point in time where I found this lump (and shared my concerns with Bruce) I was experiencing a terror that people who are lucky in life will never know and can never fully imagine.

You see, Bruce and I had already spent a great deal of time discussing how unusual it is that I do not get violently ill with the chemo. My hair is growing back. And, I seem to recover so quickly from each dose of what we have been told is mega harsh chemo. In fact, we have been told that this has been some of the most powerful chemo available . . . and it just slows me down-- but doesn't stop me.

With the appearance of a painful lump under my good arm, we were thinking the worst, and I was more scared than I have ever been in my life . . . including when the cancer was initially diagnosed. And now I was relegated to waiting to find out yet again.

Cell phones are marvelous things. They have changed the face of communication during my lifetime in unbelievable ways. They don't, however, always behave in ways that we expect.

By 3rd period, I had managed to throw myself into teaching to the point that all that my mind was registering was which students understood the concepts, and which ones needed me to present it in a different way. In other words, I was in my full teaching mode. A bizarre siren sound began from the region of my desk. It continued. I hurried to my desk, apologizing to my students on the way, and discovered that the strange sound was coming from my cell phone. (Evidently, the app from which I had applied my ringtones had ceased to function properly and the phone was now accessing an emergency signal of some sort.) It was the oncologist's office calling me back. The inclusion aide took over and I stepped into the hall to take the call.

R, Dr. K1's nurse, was not able to adequately reassure me. She suggested that I should call my local doctor and have lab tests done immediately. (It seems that having cancer crop up on the other side while one is receiving heavy doses of chemo is not unheard of.) She felt that my local doctors would be able to work me in sooner than they would and that I needed to get medical attention as quickly as possible. Upon promising her that I would call and let her know what we found, we hung up and I called my friendly local surgeon.

After a couple of months of weekly visits, everyone at Dr. G2's office knows my name. With only a couple of short bouts on telephone ignore, the receptionist suggested that I call and schedule with my regular doctor, Dr. P, since Dr. G2 was booked through the end of the week and would not be able to work me in. Upon calling Dr. P's office, they said that the earliest they could work me in would be Thursday morning. I told them that I would take the appointment offered. I then returned to the classroom and worked hard to try and get my 'mojo' back. It was much harder now that I knew I still had 24 hours before I would receive any answers. In between classes I arranged for a sub and emailed my boss to let him know that I would be out and promised to come tell him about it after my duty time during the lunch period. (Although teachers here only have duty days every eight weeks, duty time is still a pain!)

I managed to finish out the workday with a growing sense of fear and worry. My home health nurse was scheduled to come by at 5:30 that evening to check on me and monitor my vitals. (They have scaled back to once per week since the removal of my bandages. They continue to see me because of the chemo that I am on. Mostly, they monitor my vital signs and discuss with me any symptoms and/or side effects that I have.) I decided that I would show the lump to the nurse and get her take on it.

As I have told you before, one of the advantages to living in this small town, far removed from the big city services, is the rapid, quality healthcare that we have received here and come to strongly rely on. The biggest disadvantage is that I am a learning tool for most of the medical community here. Most have never seen or dealt with a breast cancer patient, so they do not know what is normal other than what they can find on the internet. Sometimes, their timing is miraculous.

When the home health nurse arrived, she brought with her some printouts that one of the other nurses had researched and asked her to deliver to me. These printouts contained information about breast cancer in very basic, laymen's terms. Receiving them while I was so worried was very helpful! I really appreciated the gesture.

By the time that I showed the nurse the lump under my arm, it was visible through the skin, and the skin around it had taken on a bruised appearance. Even I was alarmed to see how bad it looked in the mirror. Knowing that I had an appointment to see the doctor the next day reassured the nurse. She agreed that given my current medical condition, it was not something that should be put off. I promised to call the next day and let them know what Dr. P had to say about it.

Some of you are going to be upset with me by now. You will be wondering why I didn't say anything. Why didn't I let you know what I was going through? The answer is simple. Talking about it made me more nervous and jittery about what it might be. I didn't go it alone though . . . Bruce knew, and I asked my cancer survivor friends if they had ever experienced it or heard of anyone having this problem. I also don't believe in worrying others over what MIGHT be until I have answers about what IS. I'm telling you about it now.

I am happy to report that the answer to what it IS is that it is an abscess. When I asked Dr. P. how I got it, he began to talk about hair follicles. I interrupted and reminded him that I have not had any of those for a couple of months now . . . at least not under my arms. He then jokingly said that an abscess comes from bacteria. I gave him the look. He relented and said that they were very common in cracks and folds of the body . . . especially places that tend to be wet such as the underarm and under the breasts.

When I called R back to let her know, she said that she was relieved and that getting an abscess while on chemo is fairly common, but with where it chose to show up and not seeing it for herself, she was not in a position to make any educated guesses and that she would rather be safe than sorry.

The best thing that came from this week's experiences is that the home healthcare nurses have insisted that they bump back their visit time on Wednesday by an hour so that I can participate in the water aerobics classes 4 days per week instead of 3! I highly recommend it as a form of exercise . . . especially after recovering from a mastectomy!

40

Exercise Program

I am delighted to report that I have found a wonderful way to get some really deep muscle exercise that is low impact and yet feels so good! I have joined the world of water aerobics.

One of the benefits of working at Fort Stockton High School is that as a teacher here, the coach has granted me permission to use the pool in the evenings after work. In conjunction with the city Parks Department, there is from 5:00 to 5:30pm, a water aerobics instructor present in the pool. She is a delightful lady, slightly younger than my mother, who tells the most interesting stories as we work out. I have always seen photos of water aerobics classes containing students of the 'older' persuasion, so I was hesitant. Our swim coach, however, strongly suggested that it would best meet my fitness goals and that I should try it out, so I did, and love it!

Any movement in the water has always been delightful to me. While I stretch and exercise with the class, my daughter plays the mermaid in water fins; swishing her tail around the pool over and under the ropes dividing the swim lanes. By releasing the weight, while I feel light as a feather, my girl feels sleek like a fish, and we both have a grand, stress releasing time at the end of the workday.

It has taken several visits to get my courage up, but like any other recovery process, given time and patience, I finally arrived. Where have I arrived? What have I accomplished? It all started out with dressing in the dressing room (which is a typical, open high school gym dressing room).

I have been nervous and uncertain about changing in the locker room. My reasons have included uncertain feelings about how appropriate it might be for me to possibly have students walk in on me while I am changing.

Just as I wear my scarves, wigs, and hats to help the female students feel more comfortable with my bald head (It doesn't seem to matter to the boys, and I prefer just going around fuzzy headed, some of the girls appear to be physically in pain when they look at me without some sort of head cover), I have been extremely modest about my surgical scars out of consideration to them. After all, if they are pained by seeing my head with nothing on it but fuzz, how would they react if they walked in on me while changing and see my heavily scarred, flat chested side with the remaining Cyclops boob shining on the other?

This feeling of a need for extreme modesty has put me in an awkward situation more than once since I started the afternoon exercise at the pool. Allow me to describe to you what I must go through just to be able to exercise with the water aerobics class.

Water events for the mastectomy patient require specialized 'equipment'. The prosthesis that is provided by American Cancer Society is designed for everyday use. It is heavy, weighing in at four pounds. Having only a slight curve to the chest side, and covering a large area, it tends to rub even though it is contained in a 'pocket' of the bra. It also is not designed for exercise, nor (especially) for use in chlorinated water. That would break it down in a hurry and leave it pitted and not so functional. So, the first piece of equipment is a prosthesis designed for use in chlorinated water such as a swimming pool. This specialized prosthesis is designed for exercise and swimming, is much lighter than the everyday prosthesis, is completely clear, and has a hollowed underside allowing for air and sweat to pass through without as high a chance of rubbing with the exercise.

The second piece of mandatory equipment is a 'mastectomy swimsuit'. This is a suit that has a pocket for the swim prosthetic, in addition to being cut much higher so that the hole under my arm does not show when my arms are raised. This one-piece suit is a lovely black and white creation which, unfortunately, I am unable to fully put on without help from my daughter. (There is no way to pull it all the way up in the back without assistance.)

When we first began the classes, we would rush home to change. This would leave me winded and late to the class. After trying it out twice, I decided to come up with a plan to change clothes at school. For the next four lessons, I carried the box that my swim prosthesis lives in, my specialized suit, etc. . . . . I would change in the very tiny restroom stall and then, after suited, contort myself in many ways to try and 'unroll' the swim prosthesis where it attempted to fold over inside the pocket of my suit while my Zoe was pulling up on the back and under the arms in an effort to help me get the suit on properly. (I lived in fear that some curious student would open up the box and see where I had placed my bra with the form (Cousin It) still in it in the tray in the box to help 'Cousin It' retain its shape. I also was not fond of anyone who looked at the box knowing the size of my prosthetic breast because it is printed in a rather large font on the outside of the box . . . although no one who has not been fitted for one would know what it means.) In short, I decided that this method was not working for me. I set out to find a better system to prepare to de-stress and rebuild my body from all it has been through.

The next thing I tried was to wear the exercise prosthesis to work and change it over from my bra to my swimsuit before water aerobics. Because of the looser fit of the exercise boob (we named it 'Thing' in keeping with the theme started by my daughter) I decided that some of the fiberfill stuffing from the post-surgical prosthesis was in order. Unfortunately, by the time I got to work I could see that I had overstuffed 'Thing' . . . talk about well built! As my right side slid south, my left spent the day at extreme attention! (At times like this, I like to delude myself by telling me that my bald head provides a big enough distraction that no one will notice my lopsidedness . . . at least the students and staff feed my delusion by pretending not to notice!)

With some practice and creative use of stuffing and covers over 'Thing', this system seems to be working best. Juggling time does not start now until I change to swim. When I arrived this week to change, the girls from the swim team have been heavily populating the locker room, so I have shut myself into the middle stall (labeled Juniors) and done my changing from the comfort of what I am starting to think of as "my afternoon throne". Because the stall is quite cozy in its dimensions, I sit on my throne and disrobe; removing 'Thing' from my bra (being careful not to drop the stuffing on the wet floor) and carefully place into the pocket of my swimsuit after pulling my suit up to my waist. (Many times, this is an adventure because the opening to the 'pocket' is well over on the median of my left side. The challenge becomes to get it into the pocket without rolling it in the process.) I then insert my arms, call out to my daughter to close the curtain, and step out into the larger space with my scar and remaining breast barely covered, where she pulls up on the back and underarms while I juggle the front, the Cyclops, and Thing. All this is accomplished with me bent from the waist and doing something of a shimmy. (I am glad I cannot be a fly on the wall for that.)

For some reason, after suiting up, I already feel that I have done a round of aerobic exercise . . . and all I have done is suit up.

Somehow, while doing the water aerobics, I feel graceful and beautiful. Maybe it is the fact that my body is covered up by the water, the water adds grace to my movements, the instructor is very interesting and fun, and I can't see much past the end of my nose because I don't have on my glasses or contacts. I maintain that feeling right up until it is time to get out of the pool. In the water, you don't realize how hard you are working, and I am always afraid when climbing up the recessed ladder from the pool that I will not find the strength to pull myself out all of the way and will end up needing my former students who are the lifeguards to physically remove me from the pool . . . talk about embarrassing! Thankfully, just that thought tends to lend me the strength to make those legs press up through the final steps and leave the pool on my feet!

Up to this point, I had always rinsed off in the shower, washed my stubble, and kept my swimsuit on while leaving. I dried off under the air dryers . . . somewhat . . . put on a shirt over the suit and wrapped my towel around my waist. I even kept on my wet water-shoes for the drive home. Unfortunately, I have been aware that it is getting colder out. The sun has set when we leave just after 6:00 and head home. Winter is rapidly approaching. Then on Monday, in the locker room, a lovely lady who swims laps welcomed me. She had just stepped from the shower and was encouraging me to shower and change before leaving the building. I explained my excuses to her and she listened with a healthy dose of skepticism on her face. That was the trigger that helped me to take the next step . . . showering and changing before leaving.

Tuesday, due to an accident in the pool, the water had to be shocked and the pool was closed, so no class that evening.

Wednesday, the pool was again open. My instructor did not come, but I worked through as much of the routine as I could remember. I then decided to take the advice I was given on Monday and brave a shower and change back into my street clothes.

It seemed to help . . . being the only person in the locker room on this first trip to warmer travel home. I stepped in to my usual shower spot in the group shower and sank into the warm flow of water. Deciding that the shampoo I use on my fuzzy head would be the perfect gentle cleaning solution for my suit, I wore it while I took care of my hair. After rinsing, I removed the suit and rinsed it carefully. I then removed Thing from the pocket, held it under my chin while I squeezed the water out of my suit, tossed my suit on the wet floor outside of the shower and then suffered from a hefty dose of chemo brain.

I once prided myself on my quick wittedness. I now found myself with a serious case of mush brains. As I stood for what felt like a very long time under the warm flow of water in nothing but my shower shoes, I studied the prosthetic breast in my hand and wondered how I could finish my wash with only one hand. If I tossed Thing onto my towel (which was on a fairly dry place on the floor), I could not figure out how I would be able to dry myself off. If I tossed it onto the floor, I might end up with 'athlete's breast' . . . that would be HORRIBLE . . . a fate of unbelievable embarrassment!!! (I could just imagine the itching and burning on top of my fresh scars . . . and when people asked what was wrong . . . NO I could NOT go there!!!) Deciding that the only way to handle the situation was to toss Thing onto my swimsuit, I made a perfect toss. Unfortunately, Thing bounced. Just like a ball, Thing bounced. Thing landed on the WET FLOOR!!! In a panic, I leapt out of the shower and picked up Thing. (I decided that the 5 second rule must apply to prostheses as it does to food dropped on the floor.) I rinsed Thing off and then carefully placed it on my swimsuit so that I could finish my wash. (In retrospect, I will never understand why I was so worried about the contact of my prosthesis with the floor, and did not think twice about having my swimsuit and towel there . . .)

Quite proud of myself and my progress, I toweled off, wrapped myself up in the towel, and stepped into the other room with my suit to place it in the water extractor. Having accomplished that, I dressed, helped my daughter dress, and we headed home.

I am happy to report that there has been no sign of pending "Athlete's Breast".

41
Beginning Neuropathy

It is interesting to note that while today was the first day of the Christmas break (officially), it was sort of rough from my perspective.

Until this morning, I did not realize how very much I rely on work to keep my mind off of the chemo and all of the subsequent side-effects. With no work today, I find myself taking frequent naps and thinking about the various maladies that have begun to plague me with the newest rounds of the chemo. Thankfully, I will have this week and next week off and not add to the pine sap in my veins again until December 30.

Even though I had my 3rd dose of round 1 of the new chemo on Friday, being my birthday weekend had its advantages. Bruce and Zoe spoiled me terribly, and I loved every minute! My big birthday treat was a spa day at the Elegante'! I was treated to Swedish massage, a pedicure and a manicure. The staff spoiled me while Bruce and Zoe went off to do whatever Bruce and Zoe decided that they needed to do! (It was 3 hours of spoiled bliss for me!)

I seem to be having some neuropathy. This is when the chemo drugs make numb spots appear in your hands and or feet. (The numb is better than the sore.) Getting up on my feet is something of an adventure. I look like I have become very old when I first get up to walk. While Dr. K was a bit concerned about the neuropathy in my feet, he was more worried about my hands. I seem to be dropping everything (especially my keys) lately.

It can become quite frustrating to try to walk from the parking lot to the car. I noticed last week that I would drop my keys on average 3 times between the car and the school building. I am starting to learn that as soon as I reach my destination, I need to put the keys into my purse or pocket and not try to keep them in my hands. It has been an adventure to start up the engine. I also seem to drop the keys while trying to get them into the ignition. I am just considering these challenges to be part of the treatment and learning ways to work around them.

Large items do not seem to present problems at this time. Maybe I have a better 'grip' on them, knowing that they are large, or maybe I just naturally hold on to larger items tighter. I really don't know. I do know that it is becoming increasingly challenging to work with small items in my hands . . . and when I first start walking is a challenge

Back in Jr. High school Speech class, we studied how old people move and why. We spent hours practicing those movements. I even participated in a play where I was one of several 'old women' in an old folk's home. Little did I know that I was participating in a dress rehearsal for my chemo induced neuropathy.

In looking online for information on how to handle the discomfort of neuropathy, I found that one of the most highly recommended treatments is use of sublingual B vitamins. These are something that I have been using for years anyway! Perhaps I can keep my symptoms under control by upping the dose on the sublingual vitamins. It's worth a try and I will keep you posted.

42

Holiday Travels and Continuing Chemo

When we were about to turn onto our block as we headed home from chemo today, I had to laugh long and hard. (I confess that I have gotten bad about not wearing hats, scarves, or wigs during this holiday break. I find that my head sweats terribly when covered, so I am more comfortable with my fuzzy blowing in whatever breeze I can find.) When we left Odessa on our 1.5 hour drive home, I removed my hat to let the vents blow on my sweaty fuzzies. Once we reached town, I had neglected to put it back on. Upon reaching the intersection to turn off to our house, I noticed the truck in the lane next to us come to an almost complete stop. The driver was a woman who was looking at me with a look of dumbfounded incredulousness at seeing a bald (or almost bald) woman in the passenger seat of the car making the turn (me). I had to laugh. Next time I will try to remember to take a picture!

I really wish that my chemo brain did not make me think of things after the fact. Another recent incident that would have been wonderful to snap photos of was when we got ready to leave Lubbock after our Christmas visit.

We were lucky enough to be able to travel to Lubbock for a short visit during the holidays. We got to see my 94 year old grandmother (who looked very beautiful) in addition to my parents and sisters and nieces and one nephew. We also got to spend time with Bruce's sons and their families which included his adorable grandsons! (For those who think that makes me old enough to be a grandmother, know that they call us "Jamie" and "Daddy's Daddy". The grandkids also like to tell Zoe that she is not old enough to be their aunt.)

When we were ready to leave on Christmas morning, Bruce had loaded up the car while I checked to try and make sure everything had gotten packed inside. (No matter how hard one tries, there will always be items missed on a quick trip like that.) After his last trip in, Bruce informed us the neighborhood guardian had arrived to oversee what he was doing. In this case, the neighborhood guardian is a full grown tom turkey. Once Bruce had come back inside, the tom continued his inspection of our vehicle while the neighbor across the cul-de-sac tried to lure him to her house with corn.

We said our good-byes and headed out to the car. The three of us made it safely to the car although the tom did try to rush over to us for a closer look. As he came back and we hurried into the car, I was closest to him with the car door in-between us. (While he was pretty to look at, he has established a reputation for chasing anyone who visits the neighborhood. Having been chased by chickens before and pecked in the back of the knee, I did not wish to test the 'fear-factors' of being chased by a 3 foot tall turkey . . . but that is another story.)

Once we were in the car, the wait began.

Bruce had parked in my parents' circular drive with the car facing out, ready to go. The tom decided that he needed to keep us there while he inspected the vehicle. He did this by positioning himself directly in front of the car and looking over the hood at us inside. Old Mr. Turkey Tom proceeded to pace back and forth in front of the car from driver's side to passenger's side and back, but keeping his position in front of the running engine.

With the snow on the ground, I speculated that maybe he was trying to use the heat from the engine to warm himself. Whatever the thought processes of the turkey were, he was not budging from his position directly against the front of the car. I rolled my window down slightly so that Zoe could hear him as Bruce slowly moved the car forward a few inches. The tom let out a startled and loud gobble. Zoe was thrilled! We then proceeded to move forward a few inches at a time in an effort to get on the road. By now the tom was making a steady stream of comments and I believe that I am grateful that I don't speak turkey because I suspect that he was using the turkey version of sailor speak!

After several minutes of this, the old tom finally moved himself to the passenger side of the car and I let Bruce know so that he could speed up and get us out the last 5 feet of the drive without harming the neighborhood guardian! The old tom paced us explaining that he really had not given us his permission and consent to leave, but he had decided to let us pass without attacking.

We managed the rest of the trip without incident.

Today I began round 2 of 4 of the Taxol, or as I like to call it, the "Pine tree sap". Dr. K1 explained to us that over the many years of use of the Taxol for cancer treatment, it has been found that if the single dose is broken into thirds and given once per week for 3 weeks, it is more effective. Therefore, we are going with that. While round 2 began today, it will end with the third dose on January 13. That is when I will officially hit the half-way mark on the last chemo. Meanwhile, I will go back to teaching next week and back to the water aerobics (the pool has been closed for the break as well), and back to routine.

Today's chemo was interesting going in because I officially have a winter cold.

When a family is as close as ours is, it often happens that when one person catches something, everyone else in the household will get it too, no matter how hard the person who brought it home tries to keep from passing it on. (Sort of goes with the territory.) With his freezing mornings and hot afternoons, Bruce had managed to catch a cold. What he did not realize when we headed out to Lubbock was that he was running a fever. With Zoe and I closed in with circulating air while the snows fell outside, we managed to catch it too.

So, this week, I called Dr. K1's nurse to ask what I could take for a cold that would not interfere with the chemo. We discussed the symptoms and she told me that I could take anything since it sounded viral. In short, treat the symptoms and if I felt up to taking the chemo, keep my appointment. In my mind, there was no question that I would keep the chemo appointment unless they told me that I did not pass my labs. (According to many sites I have read, keeping the chemo schedule can mean the difference between beating the cancer and having it come back. One of these sites is http://www.guide2breastcancer.com/treatment/chemotherapy-staying-schedule-key-success . There are many sources online that confirm and state the increased statistics of success by staying on the schedule. You have to search for them because many sites don't want to scare you with the dramatic drop in success with misses on the chemo schedule.)

After experiencing chemo with a cold, I can highly recommend it! (Surprising, I know!) When I woke up this morning, it was somewhat better, but I was still stuffy. By the time we reached Monahans, I was 1000 leagues under water and sinking. My ears were stuffed. My nose allowed NO air in. In short, I was panting like some sort of hairless dog trying to cool itself. (It could not have been a pretty sight!) But I still pushed on for the treatment and staying on schedule. I figured that I would deal with any new side effects as they came along.

I had a new nurse today. She managed to get the port threaded properly in only 2 tries. (We have finally decided that the port sits at an angle unless I am flat on my back with my feet over my head.) The cream that they prescribed to put on when we reach Monahans works beautifully though, and I barely feel anything when they access my port now . . . it just aches after the cream wears off.

Anyway, she accessed my port and plugged me into the steroids and anti-nausea meds first today instead of Benadryl first. It was wonderful! Those steroids went to work on my swollen nasal passages and ear canals and I was breathing through my nose by the time she started the Benadryl IV!

It has been my experience in life that when I REALLY need Benadryl, it does not make me sleepy. However, if I have just a slight need for it, it knocks me out! (K-O . . . and I am down for the count . . . and as Bruce tells me . . . I sleep LOUD when I have had Benadryl.) Anyway, I don't know if it was having the steroids first, or the cold, but some combination of things succeeded in clearing my sinuses, AND I did not 'sleep loud' during chemo today. In fact, with the full house they had (standing room only for chemo buddies . . . some people appeared to have brought their entire extended families) I am proud to say that I did not sleep at all. (It was just so wonderful to breathe again for the first time all week!)

Although it was so crowded that Bruce disappeared off behind me somewhere so that Zoe could sit with me, he watched for me to sit up and start gathering things to go to the potty, and he would magically appear (my knight in shining armor) and help me to get the IV machine set so that I could move it into the bathroom with me. The one time that I did lie down for a bit, he came and stood in the area where I was receiving my treatment because he could not see my head over the half wall and wanted to continue watching over me even though he had given our daughter his accustomed place by my side. (I really don't know what I ever did to deserve such a wonderful man, but I am glad that I did it!)

This evening, I am somewhat bouncing off the walls. I seem to do alright while sitting in my chair . . . just feel like I need to type very fast. Unfortunately, my chemo brain does not let me think as fast as my fingers want to move. (That reminds me of the time that Bruce played a trick on me . . . Years ago, we had an old Apple computer with a program called ClarisWorks for the word processing. I have always had spelling issues and when I type I frequently invert letters. I automatically . . . without even realizing it . . . backspace and correct. One day, I sat down to type while Bruce was away at work. That stinker had found a way to set ClarisWorks so that every time I hit the backspace button, the machine would moo like a cow. Like Pavlov's dog, by the time he got home, I was reduced to 2 finger typing -- very slowly. It took years to get over my fear of cows!)

As I said, I am fine while sitting, but when I stand, I feel jittery all over . . . sort of like the 'jumping beans' that you used to be able to buy at the old Stuckey's roadside gift shops. For this evening, I think I will just sit here in my chair and type . . . silently!

43
Attitude Slump and Schedule Change

This feels like a "terrible, horrible, no-good, very bad day". Woke up alright, but the bad mood hit as soon as my feet hit the floor. All things considered, even in this blackest of black moods, I have to admit that I am not doing too bad since this is the first really, really bad mood since our pity party day back in July when Dr. P and Dr. G2 actually said the words, "Jamie, you have a ductal adenocarcinoma . . . that is cancer . . . and now we need to do the staging while we plan for your modified radical mastectomy (surgery).

I was not really in the mood to do anything today from the moment I got up. (That might have had something to do with waking up at 3am, wanting to go pee and having very little happen; not being able to go back to sleep and reading for an hour.) All I really wanted to do was crawl back in bed beside Bruce and dream this cancer mess away. I am tired of it. I am tired of feeling tired, and tired of the treatments. Here the end is in sight, and I sit and wallow for a while on my pity pot. We all have days like that, but I carried mine further than I needed to.

We left the house today near 7:30 to drop Zoe at school after our stop for breakfast at Donut Palace. After dropping her off, as usual, we headed to Odessa for the chemo treatment that turned out not to be.

We were concerned this morning when we arrived at the Oncology Clinic. The parking lot was unusually full, and it was almost standing room only in the waiting room. Once again, when I checked in, I wrote my $50.00 check for my co-pay and as I handed it to the receptionist, she said,

"Oh . . . by the way, you do know you owe more money, don't you?"

I must confess that I lost some of my carefully controlled composure at this point. Since October, I have been making my co-pay and having them ask me if I realize that I owe more money. When they gave me a receipt for my co-pay in November with a different patient's name on it, I started asking questions. When it happened again in December, I visited with the 'finance lady' where we discovered that my account was only reflecting $35.00 of my $50.00 co-pays each time. I was promised a full audit on my account which I am still waiting for. Needless to say, when they tell me that I owe more, my typical answer is "Oh no I don't!"

These money issues seem to be a systemic issue based on the 'money lady' telling me that she was sorry that they have not done an audit on my account yet because they have so very many patients that are in line for one before me. I feel like that says a mouthful.

Because it was close to 10am and I needed to be available for my appointment so that I would not get bumped from the cue, I rushed through my meeting with the money people and headed back to Bruce in the Lobby.

We had some items that we had ordered and had decided that Bruce would see me get started on chemo and then go to pick up our orders. When it was close to 11 and I still had not been called back for my 10:30 appointment, Bruce decided to go ahead and pick up our orders. He kissed me good bye and headed out. I was finally called back to the exam room at 11:07, but it was 12:20 before the doctor arrived and Bruce got back from his errands. (I was smart enough to text Bruce when it was nearing noon and the doctor still had not come in and ask him to pick up lunch while he was out.) I will also confess that I spent a good deal of the time I was sitting in the exam room in my increasingly worsening mood quietly letting the tears roll down my face.

I suspect that a large contributing factor in my mood is the neuropathy. That is also a huge factor in why I did not really want to get out of bed this morning.

While beginning neuropathy feels a lot like when your feet go to sleep and start waking up (as do your hands), it doesn't get better with time. The feeling just goes on and on . . . It also begins to affect the way you move, and in your hands can mess with things like typing speed and handwriting (not to mention the ability to carry things in your hands). The things that I have needed to write, like the information sheet for the doctor, show my handwriting starting to look more like my 94 year old grandmother's than mine. This morning, my fingers resembled fat sausages. (I had purchased some cheap larger sized imitation wedding rings so that I could still wear one through chemo and even those were tight on me. By the time we got home, I had to use the cold water and dish detergent to remove them because they were so tight.) If my fingers looked like bratwurst, my toes resembled Little Sizzlers.

Have you ever noticed that uncomfortable and grumpy tend to feed off of each other? They seem to do that to me when I have both at once. That is why this note is my grumpy gripe, and the next one will deal with a much more enjoyable subject . . . hopefully I will be in the mood to type it up tomorrow. But that is for tomorrow. For now, I need to finish telling you about today.

When Dr. K1 finally made it into the room, he apologized for being late. He is accustomed to me joking and he could tell that I was definitely not in a joking mood. (After I had been in the exam room for an hour waiting for him, I needed to go to the restroom, so I told the nurses where I was going. Evidently since I was not in the room when he first came in, he skipped me over and went to the next patient. He was with that patient for 46 minutes. I know this because he told me that he did not expect it to take that long.)

At any rate, we discussed the fact that I was having the numb sensation in hands and feet, and he looked at the swelling. (I sort of left out that my face and neck are swollen too, but he didn't miss that.) He told me that it looks like I am not able to handle the Taxol, and need to try the Taxotere. He told me that I am a very young woman (at least that made me laugh) and that he was concerned about quality of life issues. He said that while the neuropathy goes away in most patients, it does not in some and can become a lifelong concern. Bottom line is that we don't know which category I would fall into and he does not want to chance it since I am 'so very young.' (That earned him a second giggle.)

Bruce arrived about that time, and I recapped for him.

To make a long story short, I did not receive any chemo today. I will still have my appointment next Friday (Friday the 13th), but rather than breaking the dose into thirds, we are going to try to give me the full dose with 3 weeks break as we did with the Adriamycin. If I can handle that, I will have three doses of it and then move on to radiation. He did not offer to tell us what will happen if I am not able to handle the full dose. (I honestly hope that I am able to handle it because that would mean that I only have 3 doses of chemo left to take! Then I can start the radiation.)

Dr. K1 has prescribed a diuretic to me to help get the swelling down. I also am required to take potassium on days when I feel that I need the diuretic. The hard part will be the water intake levels that he prescribed. When I am taking the diuretic, I am told to limit myself to drinking no more than 40 oz. of anything liquid on that day. (Dr. K1 explained that he wants the medication to pull the water out of my tissues rather than out of my fluid intake and that he has found it to work better by limiting fluid intake. He also told me to expect to be very thirsty!)

When I write, I really wish that I could make it all upbeat and add in the humor I see whenever possible. Unfortunately, my goal in writing this is to possibly help someone else out with the reality of life as an unwilling member of the Cancer Club, and inform so that all of the questions that I have every day, all of the information that I wish was out there for me to find to arm myself, all of the nitty-gritty daily details of life as a member are laid out for others so that at least they can be prepared by my journey. I want this journey to mean something, and the best way I can think of to give it meaning is to put it out there where it might help out someone else who becomes or lives with another unwilling inductee into this Club.

I hope that you understand and won't begrudge me this one bad day. Overall, I think I have done pretty well so far!

44
Sex and Chemo

Sometimes it is amazing what you hear in the media! Over the Christmas holiday, while we were visiting family in Lubbock, a reporter on a newscast covered a story with the most idiotic generalization that I have ever heard in my life. What the very young female reporter said was, "People with cancer do not have sex. They are just too tired to even think about it."

I can't speak for you, but that simple-but-stupid statement hit me as wrong on so many levels. Cancer is as individualized as the people who have it. There are so many different types of cancer and stages that her comment is honestly ridiculous. Her statement was so broad that it seems to indicate that my father, husband, and ex-brother-in-law who all have had minor skin cancers frozen off would have this aversion to sex as thoroughly as a Stage IV metastatic cancer patient who was on heavy chemo and radiation with severe side effects.

This statement also does not address the individual pre-existing philosophies of the patients as human beings. Did the person have an interest in sex before? How has their partner handled the changes in the body of the cancer patient? Do they even have a partner? How does the cancer patient feel about the changes in their body? The list of questions and clarifications goes on and on.

To me the question of sex with cancer is a highly personal one, but with stupid generalizations being made in the media, I feel a need to express an opinion on this very important question. This is not a subject that I discuss with anyone very often, or very thoroughly except to crack the occasional joke. Reality sometimes causes a person to come forth with their personal beliefs and express them, however, in an effort to combat uninformed and idiotic statements . . . especially when they have been expressed in the mainstreamed media.

With cancer or without, I feel that what goes on in my bedroom is between me and the person who is with me. Sex is not a spectator sport, and it is not something that needs to be bragged about or even discussed outside of the two consenting adults who are participating in the act. (And, I am old fashioned enough to believe that it should just be the TWO participants. To me it is not a group activity either.) That being said, I will step outside of my comfort zone for the sake of attempting to correct the idiocy of the newscaster's blanket statement.

To me, physical closeness is life affirming. It is an act that demonstrates between two people that life is still there and that the deep feelings of care have not been removed with the (in my case) breast. I believe that one of the main reasons that I have been able to accept this unwanted journey so well is the absolute acceptance and support that I have received from my wonderful husband, Bruce. There have been times on this journey when it was not as easy to work around (such as the 82 days of open wounds and bandages while my body healed from the mastectomy first and the necrotic nipple second.) But, even during those times, Bruce worked hard to let me know that he still finds me attractive and loves me for who I am and not for the plaything that we had to throw away (i.e.; the 'broken toy').

Recently, while looking at a fellow cancer survivor friend's page on Facebook, I found an absolutely wonderful picture of a button (I would LOVE to be able to get one of these buttons too if I could find one). The button said, "Of course they are fake. The REAL ones tried to kill me!" There is something wonderful about knowing that you are loved in every way possible in spite of becoming an official amputee. In accordance with the sex theme question, play is also a life affirming factor. There are times when I am getting ready for bed that I will jokingly ask Bruce if he wants to play and toss him my prosthesis before boxing it up for the night. Sometimes, life is just too serious to take it that way.

Suffice it to say that while a naïve, young, inexperienced, and somewhat foolish news reporter makes an ill-informed generalized statement such as she did, at least in my case, it does not hold true.

On a different subject, yesterday's treatment seems to have gone quite well. While I was tired as all get-out yesterday and felt slightly higher up the food chain than road kill, I seem to be doing quite well today. I headed to bed about 9pm last night and slept after the treatment for the first time since this second round began. I slept in this morning too, staying in bed (between trips to the bathroom) until just after 9. Had a very nice morning snuggle too, with room service coffee in bed.

So far, the tingling of my neuropathy has lessened from what it was and the only interesting new side effect that I have noticed from this new tree sap is that my urine and other bodily waste has an interested new-growth-tree-green shade to it. (As long as my fuzz doesn't join in that green color, I will be a happy camper. I actually have enough fuzz now that when I run my hands over my head, I no longer feel scalp, just hair . . . baby soft hair.)

While my schedule has changed, I actually appear to be ahead of where I was. My next cocktail will be on Feb. 3. That means that my LAST chemo treatment should be on Feb. 24 instead of the last Friday before Spring Break. I still don't know if I will start the radiation the Monday after the last treatment, or a week or two later, but I should get that information from the doctor at my next visit. Life is an adventure. Here's to finishing chemo and safe sex!

45
The Side Effects of Chemo Medications

Step right up. Fight cancer and gain up to THREE other diseases that could be life threatening as a bonus!

In all fairness to the doctors, there are so *very many* side effects of chemotherapy that it would be difficult to remember to tell the patient everything involved with every cancer treatment. However, it sometimes seems like they forget to mention the most important points that really need to be told.

Last Friday, while I was in the chair with the Taxotere floating into my veins, the oncology nurse came over to Bruce and me and she asked if anyone had thought to tell us that the steroids that they had me take for the Taxotere cause blood sugar to go nuts. We told her that all anyone had ever said was that my blood levels "all look wonderful". She then told us that when Dr. K1 says that, he is referring to the different cell counts and only in reference to being able to take another round of chemo. She went on to say that she was bringing it up to us because my blood sugar was 'slightly elevated' at 359 and there was some cause for concern.

Some cause for concern!!! Bruce and I looked at each other, recognizing her tremendous understatement. Bruce immediately started asking questions. She told us that it was okay the week before . . . the one where they didn't give me chemo even though I had already had my steroids. It was *only* 245. With the new chemo, my required steroids were tripled and she decided that she might need to mention it to me since it was up to 359.

When we started with the chemo, Dr. K1 told us that the Adriamycin could cause severe heart problems which could show up as far away as 7 years after treatment, and many of them cause blood pressure issues during treatment, but he left out information about blood sugar.

In researching the blood sugar issues and other side-effects of the Taxotere this past week, I have found that it is also known to increase blood cholesterol levels causing later heart issues. We are assuming that they don't mention these things to you because they are trying to prevent the hypochondria factor. The general theory in the cancer centers is that what you don't know can't hurt you and unless you are a medical person, you don't need to know much. They have even told me that they don't like to share because they are afraid that it will scare me. As if.

My reply to them when we get into these 'ethical' discussions is that it is better to be informed so that I can be prepared and maybe prevent some of the side effects through advance preparations. The general answer is that they will keep me informed, but please don't use my skills as the all-time "Google Queen" and go looking for information that they have not provided to me.

This week, I went looking. The bad news about the hyperglycemia (high blood sugar) is that in studies done on the use of Taxotere, 62.86% of the patients developed it, and while only 51.26% were female, it seems to be enough of a majority that maybe someone should have mentioned it before my blood sugar jumped into the stroke range! The positive information in this study shows that the hyperglycemia was completely gone from all 62+% within 12 months of ending the treatment. (http://www.ehealthme.com/ds/taxotere/hyperglycaemia)

I think that it is safe to say that my elevated blood sugar was not the result of knowing the potential risk from the medications. (Especially since no one saw fit to warn me of the possibility!)

This week, after having talked to 2 different nurses on 3 different occasions about this issue of the astronomical blood sugar, we decided that I needed to purchase a glucose meter and monitor my blood sugar to be certain that it is caused by the medications. (Did I mention that another fun-filled, added bonus is the extreme weight gain which goes with the chemo?) The monitoring is going well. I was not able to get the monitor that I hope to have soon (it keeps the log on the computer for you by having a flash drive attachment and application that monitors and charts. I plan to order it on payday!

The monitor that I got has been rather functional . . . and very expensive! Wal-Mart did not have the test strips, so I had to buy them from a local pharmacy. While the monitor only cost me $18.00, the test strips were $126.00 for a box of 100. (Additional medical expenses are what ALL cancer patients need . . . their treatments just don't use up enough of their income by themselves!) I was unable to find any additional Lancing Drums (the drums come with 6 needles). (This is another reason that I like the other monitor. I will be able to get it, plus 100 test strips, and 100 lancets for a whopping $102 plus shipping.)

Because of the lymph nodes removed with my mastectomy, I have also needed to work left handed (good thing I am ambidextrous) to take blood samples from my right fingers only. When lymph nodes have been removed, the side of the removal requires no medical testing ever again...no blood pressure, and no needles. This is to help to prevent another medical condition called lymphedema which causes the limb where the nodes were to swell irreversibly. (I explored what happens to women who have nodes removed from both sides . . . They must take their blood pressure in their thighs, and all blood tests and IVs are done in their feet. Ouch!)

According to the 3 day chart that I kept to monitor Thursday, Friday, and Saturday shows a steady downward trend in the blood sugar. I finished last night with a 2 hour post supper measure of 149. Much better than my over 200 scores when I started the chart on Thursday. The scores seem to be the best when I get more exercise. This factor is made tricky by the peripheral neuropathy in my feet (they still tingle constantly), and the potential for injury due to their numbness. I find my best exercise to be my water aerobics on Monday through Thursday afternoons. I know that my sugar scores are still high, but they have come down so far since the start of this latest adventure.

This week has been the first Friday that I have not had to take the steroids since December 2 (with the exception of December 23 when I had no chemo). With the correlation between the Taxotere, Steroids, and blood sugar, we have done some speculating here about why things got so bad before we knew what was going on. First, I had been on weekly doses of the steroids, with two taken orally each morning of chemo on the Taxol, and followed by IV steroids prior to the chemo. Next, last week Dr. K1 had changed my dosing times to 2 oral steroids the evening before chemo, 2 oral steroids the morning of chemo, and the IV steroids prior to the administration of the Taxotere. Finally, in short, my dosage was doubled before I ever received the IV.

Bruce came up with the most logical reasoning about why things shaped up the way they have. He pointed out that the job of the Taxotere is to kill off all of the fastest growing things in my body. When blood sugar rises, my body goes into double time trying to create insulin to combat it. The chemo then kicks in to destroy all of the rapid production. (A cancer survivor that I work with, and I, were discussing Bruce's theory and we decided that it would never be proven to be true because it is much too logical.)

With another 2 weeks before I need to take the steroids again, maybe I can get this blood sugar situation back to where it needs to be. Hopefully the downhill trend will continue until it gets to where it should have been before all of this latest fun got started. If you ever find yourself in the position I am in with cancer battles, be sure to ask about how chemo and the medications that are provided to handle the side effects can work with your heart, cholesterol, blood pressure, and blood sugars. (I would never have thought to ask about the latest adventure. Just one more item on the list of things I wish I had known but no one thought to tell me.)

46
Next to Last Chemo

I knew it was a tough week at work when I found myself looking forward to chemo day. When it is less stressful to think about being told that you have blood sugar over stroke levels than to face another minute at the office, it is time to take a break. Chemo day this week was definitely worth the wait!

This week, there was a wonderful, if somewhat lonely lady sitting across from me. She was there without any chemo partner and was being given iron (which seems to be a rather lengthy and somewhat unpleasant experience from what I have seen), and she was in a talking mood. She was also a fun personality with a desire to laugh and have fun. Things really livened up when the seat next to her was taken by a good looking man who was just a few years older than Bruce . . . but still quite a bit younger than Jan, the lively lady across from me. The cougar in her came out and we were very entertained! (I never thought that a night at the comedy club drinking booze and laughing could be equaled by an afternoon in oncology being served chemical cocktails and swapping stories.) After a time, we were concerned that the folks in the other two rows were going to either demand to come join us, or complain that we were not serious enough! (It seems that too many people take cancer and its treatment a bit too seriously . . . after all, we are not dead yet, and there really is no need to speed up the process by becoming stuffy, and stodgy, and dour!)

I am afraid that my hair is thinning out again. The first clue is usually when it starts falling out from private areas. The most uncomfortable though is the nose hair . . . that and the fact that I no longer have eyebrows that are not drawn on with a pencil, and the eyelashes are a thing of the past. On a positive note, I am getting very good with eyeliner tricks! I can hide the fact that I have no lashes with creative eye makeup. (I was laughing at some of my students the other day. They were arguing over whether having no eyelashes would make you go blind. One of them was certain that it would not be possible to see if your eyelashes were to go away entirely!)

I woke up this morning composing a song in my head to the tune of "Raindrops Keep Falling On My Head". It goes something like this:

> Nose hairs keep falling from my nose.
> And eyelashes and eyebrows
> Hair from my head down to my toes
> Nothing seems to stay so
> I'm going bald again
> It's all goin' away
> But it'll be back...someday.
> Yes, it will grow back...someday...

The most positive part of this latest round of hair loss is that the hair that I have lost from my head so far is the hair of the 'lighter persuasion'. As it began to grow back last time, it was rather 'cotton like'. Bruce's youngest grandson has deep, dark brown eyes, dark eyelashes and dark eyebrows, but cotton top hair. I kept telling Bruce that maybe my hair would just be a cotton topped blonde like his young grandson. He kept telling me to keep telling myself that if it made me feel any better.

Recently, my hair has finally started to become a darker shade of blonde . . . mostly . . . and to show up enough that some of the ladies at work recently talked me into just wearing it like I do at home--without covering it with a scarf or hat. I finally did that on Thursday. I have made trips to the store and to get food without covering it up. I am starting to become accustomed to the strange looks that people give me over my nearly bald haircut. (Many seem to think that it is a style that I would have chosen for myself. I guess that I did choose it when I chose to live and fight. We can call it my crown of courage rather than my crowning glory.)

In my desire to prepare for the future and my time off, Dr. K1 graciously ordered that since my next treatment is my LAST Taxotere treatment, I will have my first appointment with the radiologist. It will allow us to put our heads together to do some needed scheduling and allow me the rest of the information that I need in order to set up what I need to set up with the Catastrophic Leave Bank at work. Of the 6 weeks that I will have daily treatments of radiation, I am fairly certain that one of them will be during Spring Break. I also want to try and schedule things so that I can be at work with my students as much as is humanly possible. They deserve as much of my time as I can give them as I go through this.

This morning when Bruce's phone decided to chirp that it needed to be recharged, I woke up to more neuropathy. This time, it seems to be hitting rather hard in the last two fingers on my right hand. At least the tingling is all that I am battling at this point in time, and not the pain that I had under the Taxol. Knowing this time that B-12 is one of the best ways to combat neuropathy, we made an early trip to Wal-Mart for massive quantities of sublingual B. On Monday, I will try again to obtain the shots from my doctor's office. While I cannot sit in his waiting room for 4 hours at a time once a week due to my current scheduling, our wonderful school nurse has told me that if I can get the shots to her, she can give them to me. I like her plan much better than the one that the doctor offered me. (My time is valuable too!)

Typing is once again an adventure . . . but just on the right side. Hopefully, with time and massive quantities of B, this too shall pass quickly. As to the hair issues . . . it will either fall out (none, some, or all), or it won't. Either way, life will prevail.

47
Last Chemo 1

All good things must come to an end, and so it is with my chemo sessions.

With the arrival of Lent, many of my students (who are Catholic) have been asking what I am giving up for Lent. My standard answer was that after Friday, I planned to give up Chemo. In one class, one of the students told me that didn't count because I was supposed to give up something that was not good for me. (I was mentally laughing at how little they understood about what chemo does to the body as a whole.) As I had my 'mental laugh', I told them, "Okay. Then I am giving up cancer!" All of the students cheered and agreed that cancer was the best thing for me to give up.

Knowing that we were to have an early appointment to meet with the radiologist for the first time and get some questions answered in preparation for the radiation treatments, I made arrangements with a beautiful teacher friend from school (thanks again, Kim Dutchover) to keep Zoe on Thursday night and get her to school on Friday so that Bruce and I would be able to stay in Odessa and be at the early appointment on time without needing to drop Zoe off at school at 6:30 in the morning.

It is VERY difficult to get weeknight reservations to any of the less expensive hotels in Odessa at this time. With the current oilfield boom, most hotel rooms are booked during the week with the workers travelling back home on the weekends. This leaves the 'one-nighters' like us in a bind. The kind lady at Best Western recommended that I call the MGM

Fun Dome and tell them that I needed the room for a medical visit the next morning. She said that they are on a published list that grants 10% discount to those who are in need of rooms due to some medical issue. Fortunately, the Fun Dome had a room available for reservation on the night needed. Unfortunately, someone forgot to tell the young lady who took the reservation that they are on that list. We were able to get a room for the night for a mere $136. (We later learned that if we will have the Oncology offices make our reservations, we can stay where they are able to get us in free . . . we just can't schedule it ourselves . . . sort of like the Ronald McDonald House does for families.)

Everything ran very smoothly on Thursday. I was really excited about this being the last chemo treatment and planned . . . then double planned . . . then planned some more. Zoe left for her adventure with Kim. (We had packed her suitcase the night before--then repacked it that morning before school when she showed me what she was thinking was an acceptable packing job. We put it in the car and had it ready after school.) I even had time for water-aerobics after Zoe left. As soon as I got home, I finished packing for us, loaded the car, and had everything ready when Bruce got home. (I am still amazed at his timing! He managed to get home right after I finished putting everything into the car!)

We headed for Odessa. Thankfully, we remembered to tell them to schedule our room for a late arrival. It was after 7:15 pm before we were able to leave home and start our drive to 'the big city'. We were still on the road when Zoe called to tell us good night and that she was being a nice guest and having a good time. We arrived at the Fun Dome shortly after we finished our call with Zoe.

One of the biggest concerns about the cost of the hotel occurred because of one of those little curve-balls that life likes to throw at times like this. While both Bruce and I were being paid through direct deposit on Friday, on Tuesday one of the rear tires on my Escape went flat, requiring me to buy 2 new tires on Wednesday. Our account balance was beginning to moan and pant. We were afraid that it would not live to see Friday.

The room was nice, quiet, and clean. I showered and changed for bed. Bruce showered too. While he was showering, I tried to put in an appearance on Facebook, but the Wi-Fi was being stubborn. I decided not to push the issue because the last time we stayed there and I pushed the issue, my email was hacked and it took me a couple of weeks to straighten all of that mess out. So I put my computer away and curled up to sleep. As soon as Bruce joined me, he set the alarm, turned off the TV, and we crashed.

My appointment with the radiologist was scheduled for 8:45, so we decided that we would get up at our usual time, enjoy the complimentary (at $136.00 per night . . . we paid for it) breakfast, and take our time in the morning.

Even taking our time, we were on the road by 7:15 am.

We arrived at the Oncology offices at 7:30 am for our 8:45 appointment. That was alright though. We had been advised to have my blood work drawn before seeing the new doctor, so we knew to plan to be there a bit early. It was interesting to learn that the Oncology office appears to be open 24 hours per day with a real, live person acting as receptionist . . . not machines and answering services. This explained to us why they have always been so good when I called on the phone! When the lady behind the desk asked if she could help us, I explained that we were there for an early appointment. She apologized and explained that the day crew would be there shortly to help us out.

We had just set our things down on a sofa when the first daytime receptionist arrived. When I saw which one it was, I had a mental internal groan.

Have you ever had a strong feeling that someone, no matter what you say or do, does not like you? That is the way that I had felt for some time about the receptionist that we now needed to face. In retrospect, I wonder if it was because the only time she would ever be cheerful was when she would wait until I had written my check and then gleefully say, "You owe more money. Will you please take care of that today too?"

To which I would generally (at least after the first two times it happened) say, "No, I don't. I have not received anything in the last three weeks that indicates that I owe any money." (After the 4th time this happened, I succeeded in getting an audit done on my account and it showed that I did NOT owe any extra money . . . yet.)

At any rate, this lady gave me the impression that she was less than fond of me.

We approached the desk to sign in with her. She stated that I was to have a 10:00 appointment with Dr. K1, and did I have my copay. I asked if there would be one copay or two since I was also scheduled for an 8:45 appointment with the radiologist. That was when everything "hit the fan". She looked at her computer screen and in a teenaged girl snotty voice looked at me and said, "Oh no, you don't."

I told her that I would get my reminder card and show her. She told me that was not necessary since her computer did not show me to have an appointment. Ever wonderful, Bruce spoke up then and told us that while we worked it out, he was going to head to the coffee pot since he had not had his morning allotment yet. That was when she looked at him and told him (in the same snotty, teenaged girl with-a-bad-attitude voice) that she does not drink coffee, therefore she does not make coffee, and he would just need to wait quietly until the other staff member who makes coffee arrived to do it.

As she was making this none-too-polite speech, the other staffer was walking through one of the doors and heading to the coffee pot. She heard how this receptionist was talking to us. She was not very pleased, and more than a bit embarrassed. Bruce, being Bruce, smiled his biggest smile at her, held out his arms as if to hug her from a distance and announced that she was now his hero since she was making coffee! Everyone laughed except for the receptionist.

I again told the receptionist that I would get the card. She said that would not be necessary and that she would "check into it". She then 'dismissed' me saying that she would call me up when she knew something. I thanked her and told her that I needed to be sure and have my labs drawn before I went back to the appointment so that I would not lose my place in the queue. She waved me away.

Coffee was made and Bruce again told the staffer (whom we had not met before) of her status as his personal hero. The waiting room began to fill with early morning patients. The nice receptionist arrived. (I call her the lady on the left. She is fascinating to watch in action. She knows the name of EVERY patient who has been there after they have been there only once and always greets them with a smile.) I was called back to give blood for my labs around 8:00 am. More people filed in. No sign from our receptionist.

Finally, at 8:15, I told Bruce that I was going to check on the status of things. I approached the desk where our receptionist was facing the wall and looking at a mail-order jewelry catalogue. The 'Lady on the left' finished with the patient she was working with, looked up at me waiting on the right, smiled telling me "Good morning, Mrs. Batson" an asked if she could help me. I explained that the other lady was helping me with a situation and I had come to see if there was any new information.

After waiting another minute or two, our receptionist slammed her catalogue shut, shoved it angrily into a drawer, slammed the drawer and told me that she was planning to call the radiology nurse and have her check her schedule to see if I was on it and someone had not bothered to put me on the central computer schedule. (I later found out that the someone whose responsibility it was to put the information from the scheduling computers onto the receptionists schedule was the receptionist I was working with.) She again dismissed me, this time telling me to 'stay in my seat until she called me'.

Either I have never been very good at following edicts from people who I consider to be paid by me, or I am taking on the characteristics of the Freshmen I teach, but I did NOT sit there until she called me. At 8:30, I again approached her. Again, after a period of being ignored, the Lady on the Left asked if she could help me this time, or was I still waiting for information. I thanked her and told her that I was still waiting for that information. After ignoring my existence again for as long as she dared, our receptionist looked at me and angrily told me that the radiology nurse had 'just' arrived and was booting up her computer. As soon as her computer was booted up and she had a chance to look at the schedule, I would be called over to the receptionist's desk and informed. I had carried my schedule reminder card with me this time and tried to show it to her. That was when she dismissed me again and attempted to instruct me to sit quietly like a good girl and await her pleasure.

I have always had a difficult time with names. In this case it was doubly difficult because I have never been given the name of either receptionist, they do not wear name tags, nor do they have nameplates on their desks. I found myself spending the next 20 minutes thinking of her name. The only fitting name that my mind was able to come up with, however, starts with 'B', means 'female dog', and rhymes with 'witch'.

Having determined that our receptionist was going to withhold any information for as long as she possibly could, and was probably the reason that every time I came to get chemo and she was the one we signed in with I was pushed back on the queue at least 3 hours . . . consistently, I waited until 8:50 am. This was 5 minutes after my scheduled appointment time this time.

Again, armed with my schedule reminder card, my wits and my dry sense of humor, I approached the desk where we repeated our drama for the audience of lobby attendees. This time, when her part was called by the Lady on the Left, she continued to face the wall and ignore me. Pushing her luck this time to the point that I was contemplating climbing across the desk and 'Gibbs slapping' her to get her attention, while still facing the wall, she angrily shouted at me that someone from the business office would come and talk with me. I asked what the nurse's schedule had shown and she repeated her shout that I needed to go sit down and wait for the lady from the business office to come and talk with me.

The new lady arrived shortly. She is the lovely, quiet, compassionate, kind lady who schedules appointments. She came to where Bruce and I were sitting (as close to the coffee pot as we could be) and proceeded to explain that Dr. K2 (Yes . . . another doctor K. It will be harder to keep up now! That's why we will call him Dr. K-2.) had a personal emergency and would not make it in that morning. He had called and requested that all of his appointments for the morning be rescheduled. I thanked her profusely for giving me real information and explanations. She also stated that since she found out what was going on, she was working closely with them to try and work me in where they could since I live out of town. I must admit that I was nearly in tears from frustration by this point and told her what had been going on in the lobby. I also lamented to her that we had spent the money on the hotel so that we would be on time and didn't really have the money to spend right now. That was when I found out that in cases like ours, we need to ask them to schedule a room for us. (Do any of you have any idea at all how very hard it is for me to ask ANYONE for help . . . ever??? I like being the one who volunteers my help to others . . . not the one who needs the help!) The scheduling lady finished our conversation by saying that she would like my permission to report the situation to the office manager. She said that another member of the staff had already reported hearing some very unprofessional comments and attitudes directed at me. She just wanted to add her story to the mix. I told her that she was absolutely welcome to tell whomever she needed to tell.

Within 10 minutes or so, we were called back to the business office. It turned out that not only was the local office manager there, but the Regional office manager was also in the office that day. The two ladies invited us into an office and asked me to tell them about what had gone on that morning. They explained to me that other staff had expressed concerns about the person in question, but that it would help them if I would let them know how I was treated by "our receptionist". So I told them much as I just told you. They apologized and told me that they will not have any unprofessional attitudes and behaviors in their office and that the situation would be addressed and corrected immediately. Then they thanked me for talking with them and told me that they were certain that if I was treated that way, so were others who might not be as willing to stand up for themselves.

Back in the lobby, before we could even sit down, my name was called to go back for my appointment with Dr. K1 (the oncologist). Things there ran smoothly. He did order an insulin shot due to the steroid induced blood sugar issues, however.

From there, we were back with the lady from the office who had been so helpful. She told us that Dr. K2 had made it into the office and that she was trying to juggle things with his nurse, J so that we could still see him and make it home in time to collect Zoe from school. We scheduled my next appointment for Dr. K1 and then she called J to come and get us to meet with Radiology.

48
Last Chemo 2

J is young, pretty and tiny. As she guided us down the hall, she apologized again for all of the problems we went through that morning. She told me that our receptionist had NEVER contacted her about whether I had an appointment, and that I did have one that the receptionist must have missed when working up her schedule for the day. (That was how I learned that it was the receptionist who was trying to cover her own mistake. She must have believed that when I rescheduled because of the personal emergency that the doctor had that no one would ever know about her mess. Guess she didn't realize that I speak teenager and it is hard to get much past me.)

Dr. K2 was very prompt in showing up. I had picked up his model of a breast that opens up to show different placements of cancer and how it grows and was playing with that while expecting to settle into a typical long wait in an exam room. He surprised me.

Upon his arrival, the first thing that he did was to apologize to me for all that one bad employee had put me through that morning. He then began to ask me about teaching and my opinions about the State assessments. It was very surprising to me because I have never met a physician who seems to be interested in what a teacher does, let alone what their opinions are about what the state is doing to their profession and the students that they serve. We discussed education for about 10 minutes.

We then went on and he began to explain the process involved in my radiation to me. Like the chemo, radiation is personalized based on type and location. He said that after the initial scans, he would have the majority of the work in determining the placement of the tattoos, and the beams and that there was a great deal of math involved.

He went on to tell me that in his experience, I would be hearing a lot of crazy stories from people sharing the misinformation that they had gathered regarding people who are having radiation.

I replied, "Do you mean like the student who told me the other day that I would not be allowed to teach them while receiving radiation because I would be too radioactive and it would endanger them?"

He laughed and told me that was exactly the type of story he was talking about. He asked me what I told the student. I grinned and told him that I told the first student who brought it up that I was just going to be transforming into Superwoman. I told the second one that he better start wearing his Geiger counter. At that, Dr. K2 and Nurse J started to laugh. I looked at him, all seriousness, and said, "I take it that they left out warnings about my sense of humor when they put together my chart."

He replied, "Indeed they did and I may have to speak to them about that!"

I love it when a doctor can be professional and have a sense of humor.

Another of the rumors surrounding radiation and cancer that Dr. K2 put to rest was the question of deodorant. Rumor has it that cancer patients cannot wear deodorant because it causes cancer. In actuality however, cancer patients receiving radiation should not wear deodorant because of the heavy rock/mineral content of the deodorant. (Look at the active ingredients on your deodorant. You will find that the primary ingredient in most is a heavy base of crushed mineral.) This tends to reflect and magnify the radiation onto the surface of the skin, causing potentially serious burns and verified serious discomfort! In answer to this, cancer centers tend to give you a recipe for cornstarch and baking soda mixed to make a powder.

As we progressed through the different experiences and expectations that were to come with this new treatment, he arrived at the point in the discussion where I was able to ask if I could continue my water aerobics. He asked what made me ask about water sports. I explained to him that in my alter-ego life as Google Queen, I found information about radiation treatments that said that swimming and any water activities would be disallowed during treatment. He smiled and told me that was the type of misinformation he would like for me to ask about. He said that I can continue, but need to be sure to rinse and wash well afterwards to remove any lingering pool chemicals, and to be sure and use lotion right after so that I don't end up making the skin dry and crack. After he finished talking about skincare, I looked at Bruce and said, "Up till now, Honey, the only thing I have had to worry about is dropping my prosthesis on the locker room floor in the gym and catching Athlete's Breast!"

That one caught Dr. K2 by surprise and had him laughing out loud. (He seemed to like the concept of "Athlete's Breast".) It never occurred to me at the time to tell him that one of my survivor friends told me that Athlete's Breast is very easy to treat . . . she said you just buy some Tenac-tit and apply it liberally!

After finishing our discussion, it was decided that we should go ahead and step down the hall for some scans so that he could start his mathematical work-up for my first treatment. J led us down the hall to another waiting room with a dressing room inside it. There she introduced us to a beautiful blonde bombshell that is the radiation tech. I was placed in the dressing room and told to strip from the waist up and put on a gown with the opening facing the front. There were lockers in the dressing room and she told me that I could place my things in there and she would hold the key while she worked with me in the scan room. I told her that would not be necessary since Bruce would need something to occupy his time while I was working with her.

When I came out of the dressing room, she was standing there waiting for me and chatting with Bruce. Bruce held out his hands. I draped my shirt and bra over his arms. I placed my jewelry in his right hand and my prosthetic breast in his left saying, "There. Now you have something to play with while I am gone." It then occurred to me that might not be the wisest idea and I told him, "On second thought, maybe not. That handful of jewelry and the prosthesis might not get along . . . not a pretty picture." The blonde died laughing.

As we walked across the hall, the blonde told me," I can't believe you said that to him! And, he didn't even bat an eye when you said it!"

The scan room is a large, open room with a curved table in the center that travels through a large, open ring. There is a form on the curved table for the patient's head, and above that, there is a tee bar for the patient to hold onto while being scanned. As you lie on the table, another cushion is placed under your knees to help keep your back aligned. After having been in there, I now know where all outer-space sci-fi movies get their engine noises for their spacecraft!

I had been well prepped mentally for the scan. They told me how to pose (sort of like going to a professional photographer . . . chin down and head tilted to the right) with my arms over my head holding on to the tee bar in a bit of a death grip. They explained that they would mark me with sharpie pens and cover those with clear bandages. (I now have a row of three bandages marching down my sternum with a fourth at the far end of my scar; nearly on my back.)

They ran the first scan with us chatting in between runs. I told them that I am thinking about getting a tattoo over my scars after I am reconstructed. Since we were discussing tattoos, after the first scan when they ran out to mark me, they opened up their sharpies and I told them that Bruce would like for it to say "Bruce's sandbox toy". Although laughing, they told me that they were limited on how they were allowed to mark their patients . . . but they would think up something special for the finale.

They sent me through the machine a couple more times and then we were done. I put the breezy gown back on for the two-steps trip back across the hall to the dressing room (Wouldn't want to scare any of the other patients with my Cycloptic appearance) and Bruce and J visited while I dressed. (Bruce had placed all of my clothing, jewelry and prosthesis on an end table rather than sitting there holding them.)

When I came back from changing, J discussed with us some of the finer points of treatment that had just been glossed over or never gone into during our previous conversation. The one that stands out the most to me is that I can still wear deodorant . . . I just need to make sure that it is one that does not contain rocks. The one that she suggested is found at Natural Foods and made of mint and lanolin. (I am looking forward to finding it. I love the smell of mint, and the lanolin will do a wonderful job as a moisture barrier.)

J escorted us to Chemo after all of that. The lady from the office had walked my chart to them while we were visiting with Dr. K2, so we knew that they should be ready for me.

When we walked into the chemo room, J told the nurse's aide that I was ready for my chemo now. The Aide glanced at the counter and told me that my chart was not yet there and that I should go out and wait in the hall. Tiny, sweet J stomped over to the desk and picked up my chart announcing loudly that it was right there and that I would NOT be sent to the hall to wait. She then told me (while they readied my chair) that I should go online and report them telling me to wait in the hall. She said that there are some patients that you would like to mess with, but you don't because that would be unprofessional, and besides all of that, she felt that I do not fit into that category of patients.

She left us when I got into my chair. The chemo nurse accessed my port with little trouble and my chemo was completed in record time.

Even with all of the extra conversations and drama, we were able to leave nearly one and one-half hours earlier than ever before. As we crossed through the lobby to leave the building, I never looked back at the receptionist desk. I did, however, tell Bruce on the way out that I might need to thank my freshmen when I got back to school. They have me so accustomed to being blamed when they are being punished because I am the one who caught them breaking rules (rather than looking at the fact that they were the ones who broke the rules to begin with) that I didn't even feel bad for the lady who probably was just fired and pointed fingers at me for being the cause!

49
Radiation and Other Types of Marks

Just my luck. Bruce had been sent out of town for CPR and extreme first aide training (training of trainers). The potential for sleep during the start of Spring Break drove away with him on Sunday afternoon.

I have never been able to sleep when Bruce is away. After 22 ½ years of marriage, you would think that I could have found ways to adjust, but it never has happened. So, I resigned myself (quietly because I don't like to worry Bruce) to sleeping poorly for a few nights.

Taking advantage of Bruce's absence with a girl's-night activities for Zoe and me, we decided to watch a movie that we had never seen before which happened to be on television that night. It dealt with a subject very close to home . . . cancer. Snuggled up together in my bed, Zoe and I watched "My Sister's Keeper". It had originally come out when Vera' and I were bald together, and Vera' drew her last breath shortly after it came out, so the timing had never been right to watch it. This time, however, circumstances were right.

Zoe and I settled in and enjoyed the movie together. She did leave for a bit when the young girl who had just started chemo again began to vomit. (That was the part she could not handle!) She returned after a while and we watched the remainder of the movie together. When it ended at midnight, I sent her off to her bed and tried some lights-out of my own.

Left to myself, I tried many things to get a good night's sleep. I shuffled pillows, rearranged bedding, etc. . . In short, I tossed and turned and felt sorry for myself because my snuggle-buddy was missing. To top things off, with all of the weather changes, my sinuses were doing a very painful number on me. I don't know how long I wallowed, but I finally made it into a fitful sleep after what seemed like hours.

Knowing that I would be getting my permanent 'spots' tattooed on the next morning must have been weighing on my mind. It led to some very interesting dreams.

The dreams began with a discussion over the available colors for my permanent inking. In the dreams, I had my choice between red and black inking. For whatever reason, I chose red. As the dream progressed through the placement and planning and marking, I ended up with a bright red grid that moved with the muscles on my chest. The grid reminded me of one used to attack the heroes in my daughter's game "Skylanders". The grid moves back and forth in an effort to hit the hero and shorten his life. In my dream, the new red tattoos did the same thing. (It was making it rather difficult for the technicians to calibrate the machine because the tattoos kept moving!)

Real life can sometimes resemble dreams. Thankfully, not entirely as the experiences at the radiologist were about to show.

After travelling to my appointment the next afternoon, once again, I found myself in a radiation room. It was a different room this time, however (nothing like the one in my dream), and it was run rather differently. Whereas last time I was placed in a dressing room and told to put on a ventilated hospital gown backwards to take two steps across the hall, this time the very sweet and very young (and very short) technician held up a teacup sized towel and told me to disrobe down to the waist. When I realized that she was holding up the hand towel to provide me with some privacy, I began to laugh . . . a lot.

It seems that the hand towel has duel functions. It provides an impromptu dressing room, and then becomes a lovely cover to afford modesty and warmth in a chilly room!

Discomfort this time reached a new all-time low. I was once again placed on a table under a machine. This one didn't have the curve to cup the back gently, however. It also had the ability to allow the technicians to pull the lower half of my body to one side and the upper half in the opposite direction. It was even able to put an interesting twist to my back which they referred to as 'leveling me out'. I was then instructed to grab the tee bar and turn my head to the right.

The tee bar sits about eight inches over the table. Arms are extended above the head to hold the bar with a slight bend in the elbows so that there is not a very deep stretch. The problem is that there is no way to rest the arms. The triceps are in constant tension during the procedure. In this instance, the procedure took about 30 minutes. (My arms are so sore . . . but I may finally get the slim triceps that I have always wanted by the time I have had all of my treatments.)

After having "assumed the position", the hand towel was placed over the Cyclops (that is what I call my lonely remaining breast) which it barely covered. The length was fine, but at my age the width was a bit more than the towel.

The young lady was joined by a young man, and the two went to work. It was a bit like being a guest in a country where you are just learning the customs and know nothing of the language. They would call numbers to each other, move equipment around me, and then call out some more numbers. Meanwhile, the towel would slip and slip and then fall to the floor. One of them would pick it up and place it back across the Cyclops only to have it begin to slip and slip again.

When the team was satisfied with their numbers, they placed the towel across my chest fully, told me to try not to move and said that the equipment would be moving in and out and might be scary to me, but not to be afraid because nothing would touch me.

After lying there with the equipment moving in and out and not moving for what was beginning to feel like a month or so, the male technician came back in and told me that he was going to be drawing on me. As soon as he took the lid off, I recognized the odor of a Sharpie. True to his word, he began to trace.

With nothing to move but my eyes, I began to observe the process. Inside the large, round lens of the machine there exist many metallic looking slats. These moved into different positions depending on where the machine was aimed. Light shined on me where these slats were opened in interesting geometric patterns. It was these patterns that the male technician was tracing on my body with the sharpie. At one point, he managed to trace over the tickle spot under my arm which nearly caused me to have convulsions. (Having not grown up ticklish, it still takes some getting accustomed to when it is touched.) Since I was still not allowed to move, I had to settle for a good scream. The young man used a more careful drawing hand after that.

As I lay aging on the table, the two technicians continued speaking in numbers, leaving, coming back, and drawing only to repeat the process again . . . and yet again.

Finally, I was told that they were finished with that part and it was time to get my permanent tattoos. Still not allowed to move, the young lady talked me through what she was doing as she marked me. She painted on (or at least it felt like painting on) the ink, then told me as she was inserting a needle to assist the ink in getting under the skin. I almost felt nothing on my left side where I still have numbness issues from the surgery, but I really did feel the one that was placed under my arm on my right side. (They said that it was a mark to assist them in 'balancing' me.)

The young lady has very good vision, but has obviously never seen freckles. She told me that the spots that were being inked on me would be about the size of a freckle. When I manage to find one, a blackhead inside of a very small pore is what comes to my mind. I now have four permanent blackheads on my left side, and one on my right. I will have them for life.

When I looked into the mirror after being helped off of the table (the technicians had to help me lower my arms. I was unable to move them) I caught a glimpse of myself in the mirror in the room. There I stood, holding a tea towel over my chest with black Sharpie drawings from the base of my ribs to my jaw line on the left side. The technician was telling me that I could leave, but I was having a laugh attack at the thought of the stir I would cause walking with my daughter into Jason's Deli with the very prominent Sharpie marks. After I was able to stop laughing and catch my breath, the technician helped me to try and wash off the marks with the small square alcohol swabs. (It only took us about 30 each, and then my skin was fairly blue from the ink.)

Today was my first official treatment. I should have a total of 33, so I now have 32 to go.

Zoe and I slept in this morning. (I actually slept well last night. I do wonder if that is a blessing of the Tamoxifen . . . the hormone medication that I will be on for the next 2.5 years that is designed to starve the cancer cells by denying them estrogen and/or progesterone in my case. At any rate, the sleep was much needed and very much appreciated!) That translates to us sleeping until about 8:00 am. We headed to bed early too last night. We must have been asleep by 11:00!

Fresh from good sleep, we ate breakfast at home, and picked up some burritos on our way out of town. (Mine was brisket, hers was bean and cheese.) We travelled a different route to Odessa today and found ourselves there much earlier than we had allowed for. This being the case, we decided to stop at Family Dollar and get some cheap lipstick on our way to the Cancer Center.

When we left Family Dollar after making our purchases, as we were getting into the car, a young man came running out of the store and calling, "Excuse me . . . excuse me, Ma'am!"

Zoe had already gotten into the car and closed her door. He approached on my side of the car and I kept my driver side door between us. He was young (about 25-30 years old), clean cut, about 5'6" and slim to medium build. He came all the way to my open driver's door and asked me if I knew where some apartments were. I told him that I was from out of town and didn't know where much was. He then began to grill me with questions . . . trying to get me to tell him where I live, specific address (I was deliberately vague, but told him that we were from Fort Stockton. Then he started in about having relatives here and where exactly did I live. He mentioned the main street in town and asked if I lived near it. I told him yes since I figure that everyone in town lives near that main street!)

As he tried to throw flattering shinola my way, he kept looking at my purse. He finally decided that I was not going to volunteer any personal information or move from behind the safety of my car door. That was when the kid asked me if I was married. I told him that yes; I am very married and very happy that way. What he said next floored me.

As this young man (my step kids are older) was trying to get personal information from me, all I could think about was the physical reality of who I am at this time in my life. I am a 49 year old woman who is just starting to get my hair back. I am carrying around an extra 30 lbs from chemo that

I didn't need before I had the chemo and which seems to be emphasized by my lack of hair to hide it. I have rolls and lumps where I used to be flat, and a large flat scared spot which is covered by artificial rolls and lumps which once had real rolls and lumps there. Whatever he was selling, I was not buying . . . especially when he apologized and told me that he really just wanted to get to know me because he thought I was really 'hot' . . . in fact . . . 'smoking hot'.

Dealing with teenagers on a daily basis, I have a very well developed nose for B.S. and other types of bodily wastes. Suffice it to say that my 'crap-o-meter' was buzzing on full-of-it stage. The young man then ran for his car and, after he wrote down my license plate number, he took off.

As I got into the car while the young man ran away, Zoe looked at me in a very disapproving way and said, "I heard that whole thing."

We went on to the Oncology office and I tried to forget about the whole incident (after having explained to Zoe that I had not done anything for her to be mad about).

Once again, my arms wound up sore. Today was the real deal. It ran much like the practice from yesterday . . . including the use of the tea towel for 'modesty'. The one variation in the process was the addition of a Geiger counter wire to measure my last dosage for the day and assure the staff that I was receiving the right amount of radiation exposure. (Such a comforting concept!)

The most reportable aspect of today was that I could not get the incident at the Family Dollar off of my mind. As we left the Cancer Center, I spotted the Police Station. We went in to let them know about a young, crazy man hitting on rather bald women with cancer. The clerk there tried to assure me that I was being most helpful since there is currently a group working in the Odessa area who are praying on 'older folks'.

Some days it doesn't pay to try to be a good citizen!

50
The Rhythm of Radiation

I am falling into the rhythm of the radiation treatments. I have even learned how to power nap on the hard tables. There is a certain pattern that is followed with most visits and it is rather comforting in its predictability.

Mondays are doctor visit days where I actually have a standing appointment with the doctor so that he can examine my skin for radiation reactions, and to learn of any other concerns that I may have or problems I may be experiencing. In addition to this standing appointment, I have "skin days" which are the days when the machine is tricked into not sending the radiation as deep. Let me explain.

On skin days, rather than just the usual tea towel (which I have been informed is actually a highly starched pillowcase . . . my response to that was that my one remaining pillow is larger than their case) a clear, one cm thick silicone sheet is taped to my skin where the radiation is to be given. (It is warmer cover in the cool room, so I really do appreciate skin days.) This false skin is used to 'trick' the machines into just skimming the surface of my real skin with the radiation in order to be sure that the surface of the skin does not harbor any cells that are cancerous. They tell me that it is especially important over the scar tissues because cancer has a tendency to recur in the areas where previous cancers have been removed. (Since this is the statistical finding, extra care is made to ensure that my lymph glands are covered too, including those in the left side of my neck, because four of the ten that were removed were positive for cancer.) Skin days just take a couple more minutes than regular days, so that is not a problem. Dr. K2 has prescribed them for me every third treatment.

As we have progressed through the radiation, I have noticed that in some ways I preferred the chemo to the radiation. With the chemo, the pattern of side effects was more drawn out with a greater time for feeling like there was some recovery. With the radiation, I feel decent when I wake up, but within 30 minutes of the treatment, I feel like a pork roast with the oven set on broil. Bruce has compared my poor underarm with the burns so many of our generation got before we knew the damage we were doing by lying in the sun. People would suntan using baby oil with iodine and get a ferocious burn and peel. I have that level and look of burns under my arm (an area that I highly advise against burning) just without the peel yet. So far, I have used ½ of the bottle of 100% aloe vera that Bruce bought, and still have 15 treatments to go. (At least that is more than half-way done from the 33 treatments that I started out with!)

On my first skin check visit with Dr. K2, standing in his exam room beside him in my ventilated night gown as he said, "Let's take a look", I looked him in the eye and began.

"Before I do this, you need to know that you are about to join some elite ranks. Aside from my husband and my daughter, the only people to whom I have shown my scars include . . . your entire staff, the entire staff of PCM Hospital, the entire staff of PCM Clinic, and the entire staff of PC Home Healthcare . . ."

Before I was half-way done with my list, he was laughing out loud. He (rightly) summed it up by stating that I was having some privacy issues (changing in an open room with cameras behind a tea towel . . . you think?). He apologized on behalf of his profession. He said that sometimes they get so caught up in the job that they forget the sensibilities of the patients for whom they are doing their job.

I was very impressed with is candor and his attitude.

I had a really big scare on the first day of the third week. That Monday morning, when I got up and was getting ready to go teach, I looked in the mirror and saw hundreds of small scabs under my arm. They were all loose, and some were clusters of hair held together by scabs. When they tell you that you will lose your underarm hair, you lose it; just not the way you expect it to go! I was glad that it was doctor day so that I could get more information about what was happening.

At the time, he told me that we would take a couple of days off of the treatments to the underarm. I guess he changed his mind because no time was taken off and my orders were not changed to reflect what he had said. I do not know if that was because he had a substitute for his nurse, or if he changed his mind, but I will definitely be asking about it tomorrow.

One of the nicest things that has come from my treatments is getting to know the people on the staff in the radiology department. The buxom blonde that I mentioned to you earlier is a cancer survivor. She loaned me her copy of <u>Why I Wore Lipstick to My Mastectomy</u> by Geralyn Lucas. It was a wonderfully written reflection on going through breast cancer from the perspective of a 28 year old. I found myself comparing and contrasting the differences and similarities in attitudes between the 28 year old perspective and my 48 year old perspective. I also noted things like geographical distances . . . she travelled by taxi to her treatments; I drive 1 ½ hours to receive a 15 minute treatment, then travel back again. The one thing that will probably be with me for the rest of my life though is that I cry real tears at the happy ending.

With the burns under my arm getting so seriously bothersome, I talked with my Principal and the counselors at school about things last Monday. My prosthesis weighs four pounds. Its rubbing on the burned scar tissue was beginning to feel rather 'harsh'. Together we determined that the time was rapidly approaching when I would need to leave 'Cousin It' in its box and make my way without company for the Cyclops.

If I were not so well endowed, it would not be an issue. I find myself frequently brooding about the fact that the Cyclops is so large . . . still a triple D on that side. Wishing that I had been able to convince the surgeon to do a bilateral operation, but being unable to does not change the reality of my situation. It is rather difficult to conceal the asymmetrical state of my body these days. Bright patterned shirts tended to disguise the size discrepancy, and gave me an excuse to go shopping for some camouflage, but I needed to prepare my students too. (I could just see me not mention anything and then have them all stare at the Cyclops while I am trying to teach them.)

After my discussions with the powers that be, I began each class by thanking them for their patience and support as we have gone through this journey together. I then explained my dilemma. (There was at least one student in each class who had no idea that I wear a prosthesis, and another who would invariably ask 'why' I need a prosthesis . . . to which the other students would ask, "Where have YOU been all year?")

As I explained the situation to them, most were understanding. I explained to them that we humans find symmetry pleasing to the eye whereas something asymmetrical draws our eyes like a bad car wreck . . . we want to look away, but we just can't help ourselves! I went on to tell them that I was filling them in on the situation because I was going to need to start leaving the heavy sucker at home and why. I went on to say that when you know you are about to pass the wreck it might be easier not to stare, but that if I did not let them know in advance I was afraid that I would be standing before them trying to teach and find myself to be that car wreck . . . and that I was not comfortable with that idea . . . I would prefer that they treat me as normal. (At least as "normal" as I ever am . . .)

After power shopping that afternoon, I arrived the next day with only the Cyclops and camouflage. Only 4-5 students in my first period class noticed. (It was almost laughable to see their faces when they realized that I was using smoke and mirrors.) They politely looked away and did not say anything. One or two noticed in subsequent classes, and so I made it through the day.

I found that wearing the prosthesis and the pain from it rubbing was causing me to be very tired. Not wearing it perked me up considerably even though I remain very self-conscious about how flat it is compared to how large the Cyclops is. Strangely, it is the Cyclops that I find myself resenting rather than the lack of a breast on my left side. This causes me to wonder if I am mentally as normal as I like to think that I am.

51
Some Days are Like That

Never ever, ever sunburn your armpit!

Radiation burns under my arm and those along the side of my neck became really bad. The skin was a rather deep purplish-black. At my doctor visit for skin check, he rearranged my schedule to have my 'boost' treatments moved up. (Boost treatments are those that concentrate highly on the scar tissues since research and time have shown that the surgical scars are one of the favorite places for cancer to return.) This change places my last six regular treatments on the end.

My last boost treatment was today. I will miss them. They only took 30 seconds once the table was set up. That left me driving for an hour and a half to a 30 second treatment followed by another hour and a half drive home in time to pick Zoe up from school. I have managed to learn all of the new songs out on the country music stations and can sing them quite well!

Due to the events of this morning, I have been given a three day weekend from the treatments.

One of the first lessons that you learn about having cancer is that life still goes on. Our landlord contacted us last month and told me that he promised our house to his brother and that we need to move out sometime this summer. Yesterday, we finally found and committed to our new location. We will start our move after the 15th of next month. That puts us in the prepping to move mess right now. It makes life interesting . . . and keeps it that way.

The politics of work also jump into play in my past week and a half. I ran out of personal leave time. I had, up to this point, managed to continue working with my classes in the morning, and heading to my radiation in the afternoons. The day that I ran out of my personal leave time, I received notice that I could only receive benefits from the Catastrophic Leave Bank if I was off full time. In short, if I worked ½ days, my salary would be docked ½ days. If I stayed off full time, I will be paid full time. Needless to say, I am off full time now. I really miss my students!

Being off full time does allow me to run errands in the morning, and do things like cleaning out my closet in preparation for the move. Yesterday, I donated 66 gallons of clothes. (I figure that there were 66 gallons of clothing since I used two full 33 gallon bags!) Because I still don't know what my final shape will be when all of this fun is over, and I don't want to move a bunch of clothes that don't fit, I managed a very thorough cleaning of my clothing stores.

This morning, in preparation for our move, I was going to run out and check on some things that we needed. With the extra time on my hands, I am the logical candidate. My instructions from Bruce are simply that I should not overdo things. (Easier said than done!) My plan was to just run, be back in about 30 minutes, and come home with time to do a couple of loads of laundry, wash some dishes, and tidy up the house a bit. (I had already taken out most of the trash.)

With the plan firmly in mind, I grabbed my purse and keys, and made an on-the-spot decision to simply lock the knob on the front door since I was only going to be out for maybe 30 minutes. As the door swung shut with a bang, I realized that I had grabbed the wrong set of keys. In my hand were the keys to the school and my classroom. Locked safely inside of the house were the keys to the car and the house. Sadly, we had recently increased the security of our home due to an incident earlier in the week.

Last Monday morning while getting ready to take Zoe to school, I stepped into her room to turn off her television and noticed that I could hear the birds singing as if they were in the room with me. Concerned, I pulled her curtain back just a bit and discovered that her window was open just under an inch. It was open just far enough to not trigger the alarm.

Since my girl was in the kitchen making her lunch for school, I quietly stepped outside and around the corner of the house to look at her window from the outside. What I found there scared the crap out of me!

It was obvious that the screen had been loosened from the outside. Two of the screws were only partially in the screen. Two more were on the window ledge.

I went back inside and did my best to close her window.

After running her to school, I ran up to the high school and returned graded papers for the sub to pass out and left her the lesson plans for the week. I also needed to be on campus to save them to the staff drive on the computer so that they are accessible to the administration and special programs that need them. (I later found out that when I was told to go on full leave, which also means I must find other ways to make those exchanges. I am not supposed to be on campus at all.) As I left the building, I saw our campus policeman and asked his advice about the window at home. He promised to come by and photograph it in case something else happened later on.

When I had already run myself to exhaustion after returning from my regular Monday radiation routine (including the doctor's skin check), I made one more run; this time to the local hardware store, and bought a ¾ inch diameter dowel for Bruce to use as another lock on the window. He had already stated that he planned to get home before dark so that he could get all of the screws back into the screen.

Needless to say, after all of the excitement of discovering the open window (which none of us had opened), we were being very security conscious. Especially when Bruce discovered that the screen had been removed completely and the reason there were screws not completely in was that the perpetrator had tried to put the screen back on and done it upside down . . . the fact that they were trying to cover their tracks was as scary as anything about the situation, and we became hyper-vigilant. (Remember. . . this was the window to our little girl's bedroom!)

Sometimes it doesn't pay to be quite so careful to keep everything locked up.

I found myself, as I said, outside with the important keys inside and the door locked . . . on the hottest morning of the year so far. (When I passed the Dairy Queen in Odessa at 1:00 as I headed to my radiation appointment, their sign said 103 degrees.) Thankfully, I had my cell phone, and the car was not locked so I was able to sit somewhere other than the ground. (My wonderful neighbor offered me sanctuary should I need it, and though I needed it desperately, I was determined to get into the house!)

I began calling. I know that the landlord's handyman has a key. I called his number, but was sent straight to voicemail . . . so I left a message. I then Googled locksmiths in the area. There was one listed who, as it turns out, was and is the only one in the area. Unfortunately, I found out later that he did not answer his phone or cell because he broke his hand and was at the doctor. Bruce texted me back and suggested that I contact Zoe at the school and get her key. (When I got Zoe on the phone, she told me that she had taken her key out of her backpack and it was somewhere in her room.) I called the officer from school and asked him if he had any ideas.

To make a long story short, the wonderful officers from our police department helped with creative thinking and after a long time and quite a bit of work, we were able to get in. In all, I was locked out in front of my house for about 3 hours.

One of the first instructions you are given when you start radiation is to avoid spending much time in the sunshine. While treatments are still in progress, the skin is especially sensitive . . . even under clothing. While this hypersensitivity is reported to continue for life, it is especially heightened during treatment time and for the first year afterwards. Three hours in the morning light was not kind to me.

Currently, my least favorite activity is sweating. You see, just like with sunburn, when you sweat, blisters show up. When blisters show up, they pop. When they pop, the skin becomes weepy and peels. After three hours in the morning sun, I was sweating.

When I got back into the house, I had 30 minutes to cool off before I needed to make my long drive. My tickle spot no longer tickled. And, the areas where I had very little feeling since the surgery now had feeling . . . and it was not pleasant.

By the time I got to radiation, the blisters that had developed over the morning activities had all burst. The majority of my scar line was weeping.

The peeling hole under my arm was weeping. Most of the dead and burned skin from my armpit was peeled, peeling, or about to peel and weeping. Any movement of my pectoral muscles was very uncomfortable. On the closed-circuit TV screens, the technicians must have seen the tears that rolled silently down my cheeks from the pain of the 30 seconds holding on to the T bar. My ticklish spot does not tickle any more.

Thus, my orders were to take a long weekend and allow some healing. On Monday, the routine is to be reversed . . . Dr. K2 is to look at the skin first and then decide if we can get back on schedule with the last 6 treatments. That is how close we are to the finish. Maybe, if I can be very, very good, maybe I will be able to finish up only one day late.

52
Stupid Questions Deserve Obvious Answers

There comes a time in every cancer survivor's life when they are tired of filling out forms for the latest new doctor. As a teacher, I often want to just shout at them all, "Can't you fools just share!!!" Of course, I know that will never happen, so I usually play along just like the rest and be good.

I suspect that I reached my 'be good' limit before I ever got that enormous packet in the mail from the office of the plastic surgeon I am supposed to meet tomorrow morning. (Filling out the medications alone will be akin to writing <u>Gone with the Wind</u> or <u>War and Peace</u> . . . nothing short of a classic novel.) At least the papers were mailed to me so that when the humor breakdown occurred, it was in the privacy of the restaurant we were dining in and not in the middle of the doc's waiting room where people who don't know and understand me might think that I was in the throes of a mental breakdown. (That is how bad my giggles got to be.)

In all fairness to whomever it was that wrote the forms, they worked very hard to try and word their questions in enough of a generic manner that they could be used for any manner of surgical solutions. (It seems that this surgeon wants to be thought of as a surgeon first and the 'plastic' part as secondary.) All I can say in my own defense is that I am tired. After nine months of being identified as a 'breast cancer patient' as my primary identity, and having the majority of my conversations with friends and strangers alike being centered on my current prognosis and treatment, I am tired. I am bloody tired of the whole mess . . . Unfortunately, it will continue for many more months. (I really doubt that you will blame me for being tired of it all . . . I am sure that you are rather tired of hearing about it too.)

These are the thought processes that were going through my head faster than the speed of light when I got to the two questions in the book that the doctor's office asked me to fill in . . . and they were my undoing.

The first question was not too terrible (although I am fairly certain that no one will ever read my answers since they tend to have you write all of this mess for your files and then they ask you the same questions again in the visit and write it all down again). It was, simply stated, "REASON FOR VISIT". At this point, every story I have ever heard or read came into my mind . . . along with thoughts of Barbie dolls and every blonde joke (I admit it--I love blonde jokes--Like Aggie jokes, they are good advertising for those of us who were born blondes!)

I managed to pull my imagination back in check and wrote "Reconstruction after breast cancer".

The question that followed was the one that was my undoing. I read it and the giggles started because I could only think of one possible answer to the question. The question was, "WHAT SYMPTOMS ARE YOU HAVING".

In retrospect, I could have listed the lack of eyelashes and eyebrows unless I draw them on. I could have gone into the peeling skin and burns from the radiation, or explain that I had to have my port flushed just today to "keep it happy". I could have explained the surgeries, the tumors, the hell of having the diagnosis of cancer. I could have done any of those, but they didn't enter my mind at the time. The only answer that I could think of to the question, "WHAT SYMPTOMS ARE YOU HAVING" was to write, "I woke up on August 2 and my left breast was gone." (And the giggles hit me again.)

I wonder if this doctor surrounds himself with people who understand using humor to cope, or if it will be those who have no sense of humor and disapprove of those who do. I guess that I will just go to the appointment tomorrow and find out for myself.

53
Healing Time

God has a sense of humor.

I have known for many years now that God has a sense of humor and he seems to appreciate all opportunities to share a laugh if we just stay sharp enough to recognize and appreciate the jokes. (Often, the jokes are on us, or we are part of the jokes. At least that has been my experience.)

Lately, I find myself puzzling over the great cosmic question. My question is not the traditional question about 'why we exist', or 'what is the meaning of life'. My question is whether my sense of humor is a reflection of God's sense of humor, or does he temper his sense of humor to meet mine to enhance my understanding. For me, that is the ultimate cosmic question.

It has been an interesting few weeks. I still have been unable to take my last three radiation treatments because of the severity of my radiation burns. Because of the burns, Dr. K2 will not release me to return to work. With only two weeks of this school year left, I am feeling rather conflicted. It is pretty hard to send lessons, grade papers, and not have access to the students. I miss the students terribly, and feel like I am cheating them out of what I should be able to be there and offer as far as my ability to help them on their educational journey. (Dedicated teachers, like me, seem to have this ego issue that screams out that no one, no matter how wonderful, can give the students exactly what we can.)

The healing process from these radiation burns has brought back unpleasant memories from my 82 days in bandages after the mastectomy. One of the hardest hit areas is the scar tissue over where the seromas were back in the fall. The weeping and mess reminds me a great deal of that time. The issues with tape have not changed either. Even the super mild paper tape will grab hold on my skin and remove the hide instantly, leaving additional sores to deal with. Fortunately, it appears that the wounds are healing well enough that possibly this next week will finish up my last three treatments (finally). However, with this in mind, most days are spent in a condition that I would not want my students (or anyone else for that matter) seeing me . . . topless.

As a young girl, I once thought it was terribly unfair that boys could take off their shirts and go topless whenever they wanted to, but it was unacceptable for girls. Now that I am 49 and have those social mores firmly entrenched as the societal norm, I find that I have spent the majority of the last four weeks topless. This has allowed my burns to 'breathe'. As a result, I have tended to keep the curtains drawn, the doors locked, and a shirt close-by. Much of the time is spent napping. I have convinced myself that this is my body's way of trying to heal.

Last week, we had three days of rain. Bruce came home just after lunch on Thursday. Because his truck was acting up, he decided to use his time working on the engine. Naturally, he opened up the garage door to make access to his tools easier.

Our door that leads from the kitchen into the garage has a large glass window in it. Because the external garage door usually stays closed, we have never put a curtain or shades on it. With my usual sitting spot where I have my laptop and general recovery area set up facing the garage, I have never felt uncomfortable about the uncovered window because I never open up the door to the outside.

With Bruce home and working on his truck, I sat myself in my typical topless pose and played on the computer for a bit before taking a nap. Bruce came in and woke me to tell me that he was heading to the parts store for materials to continue working on his car's engine. He told me that he had locked the doors since I was having my 'topless time'. What he didn't do, however, was close the big garage door. Meanwhile, he left and I resumed napping.

About 30 minutes later, sleepy eyed, I woke up and glanced at the TV. From the corner of my eye, I saw a man moving about in the garage. In a topless panic, I grabbed my pink Harley cap from the back of the sofa and through the Cyclops inside! (It is sad when your one remaining breast fits into your baseball cap better than your head does!)

With the Cyclops safely hidden in the baseball cap, I ran for the back bedroom to get a shirt to cover more properly.

Since all of this started, I have had horrible thoughts of a student inadvertently seeing my scars and winding up scarred for life mentally by the image. It is totally irrational, I know, since being seen by my husband and daughter on a daily basis does not bother me. The home health nurses never left the house screaming after any of their visits, and the ladies at the water aerobics classes never balked. Maybe I am really more concerned with people seeing the Cyclops than I am with the scars . . . after all, the Cyclops is rather large and scary.

Long story short, the man in the garage was Bruce. He had returned home and forgot to let me know.

One of the areas where God's sense of humor has become most apparent is my hair. All of my life, I have thought it would be nice to have curly hair. I have thought so to the extent that I have prayed about it from time to time. Unfortunately, I have not been specific enough in my requests. I now have curly hair for the first time in my life. It is the new hair that is growing in and replacing my right eyebrow. (Not exactly what I meant when I asked for the curly hair, but I was too generic in my request. Next time I know to specify that when I talk about the hair on my head, the exception will be my eyebrows.) As to the rest of my hair, it all grows to the left. Every hair on my head is growing to the left. Thank goodness short, side swept hair is in vogue at the moment.

Another problem with my hair has been the color. In doing some online research, it is most common for the hair to come back in either jet black or grey with very little variation. I have not enjoyed having more grey in my hair than my mother who is in her 70's! The final straw was yesterday when the landlord of the house we are moving into next week came by. My daughter happily answered the door. She died laughing when he asked her if her grandparents were here. (I didn't find it so funny, personally.)

While my mother has tried to convince me that dying your hair is time consuming and a lot of trouble, I find that it is no different than giving yourself a deep conditioning treatment every other month. With that in mind, Bruce and I headed to Wal-Mart where I had him select the new color that I determined (after more internet research to be sure that I had waited long enough to prevent any wild colors from forming) it was time to have. I must admit that my daughter was very disappointed afterwards that my hair did not turn orange, purple, green, or some other equally inappropriate color.

My visit to the plastic surgeon was somewhat disappointing. He was very unimpressed with my radiation burns, and I suspect that when I go back again at the end of June that he will advise me to wait at least another year before I begin the reconstruction process. He has stated that he will not use an implant. He is afraid that with my allergies and the condition of my skin that my body would reject an implant and that within one to two years, it is possible that my body would push the implant out through my very damaged tissues. (Gross when you think about it . . . the stuff of nightmares!)

The only type of rebuild that he recommends for me would be a tram-flap operation. The damaged skin would be removed completely and the skin and fat from my stomach would be moved up to build the new breast. In short, I would receive a tummy tuck along with the breast rebuild.

All of this is dependent on how much my skin heals between now and the end of June when I go back to see him again. Meanwhile, the Cyclops and I will keep hanging out and healing.

54
Celebrations and Confessions

We have arrived at a time for celebration and reflection.

I finally finished my last radiation treatment yesterday. It was a long, hard road, but I reached the goal and completed the recommended treatments and the recommended number of treatments. The beautiful, buxom blonde in the radiologist's office who originally initiated me to the world of radiation treatment was the one who presented me with a frame-able "Certificate of Merit and Appreciation". It says, "Be it declared that Jamie Batson has completed the prescribed course of radiation therapy with the highest degree of courage, determination and good nature. We appreciate the confidence placed in us and the opportunity to serve you." It shows to be from the Oncology offices.

The battle was a long, hard one. While I have always worked to put on a brave face in the face of adversity, I can honestly say that I breezed through the chemo but the radiation nearly killed me! At one point, after I was forced to go on full time leave from work, Bruce was worried that the burns were bad enough that we might need to consider hospitalization. He was afraid that he was seeing my bones where the deeper blisters had popped and were peeling and weeping. Had I been able to stay on schedule, treatment would have been completed April 27 rather than May 31.

You might ask yourself why I kept on until I had gotten the full course in spite of the astronomical amount of damage sustained by my skin. The most direct answer would be fear.

I must be a reincarnation of Cleopatra because I have been operating as the undisputed queen of de-Nile. I believed that if I kept it light, the reality of how serious things were would not touch me as deeply. To a large extent, my theory was right. As I sit here now facing the great wait leading up to the next set of scans, I find myself in the unenviable position of facing my cancer head on.

No jokes. No humor. Nothing to look at but straight facts.

The first tumor showed up in one week. By the end of the next week, there were three tumors totaling over 7 cm. Pathology showed them to be the highest grade that they could possibly be. (This means that they were as fast growing as they could possibly be with as terrible mutations as they could possibly have, too.) During my modified radical mastectomy, they found four of ten lymph nodes positive for cancer, and one of these lymph nodes had a "thread" of the cancer shooting out from it and imbedding into the muscle wall of my chest. (That is the little detail that I managed to keep from you until now.) I was a high grade Stage III on the verge of becoming a Stage IV with metastases.

I was never told at the time, but recently learned that I developed blood clots in my legs while undergoing the mastectomy surgery.

On the most positive note, I tend to be as tough as an old boot. According to my oncologist, Dr. K1, all of the surgical margins were clean and clear and free from cancer cells. We went through the chemo because if we had stopped after the surgery that 'got it all', I had a 98% chance of it all coming back. Chemo took that down to around 75% chance of it coming back. The radiation (all agreed that this was the most important part of the treatment) reduced the chance of recurrence to 10%. He stressed to us that I am to consider myself to be a survivor who went through treatment to prevent it all from coming back.

From this point, I will be on Tamoxifen for the next 3-5 years. (Dr. K1 says that he will consider changing me to a newer hormone therapy after 2.5 years so that I can have a couple of years of 'different' side effects.) The primary side effect that I have noticed from the Tamoxifen is that I break a sweat like a racehorse after running the track twice every time I get up and walk for 5 feet.

My biggest problem right now (other than too much time to think too seriously about this past year) is that the ankle I injured during our move is actually broken even though the emergency room doctor told us that it was only a sprain. The prognosis for my "fractured fibula" is good; projected healing time is 4 weeks more rather than the 8 weeks or more that a sprain could be. The biggest problem has been how to keep me off of it.

Crutches were the first recommendation from all 3 of the doctors who have seen me about my ankle. Unfortunately, crutches are out of the question. The new skin under my left arm and across the scars on my chest is too new and fragile to handle crutches. My cane does not remove enough weight from my leg, so I am the proud renter of a wheelchair and a "get about". I am having fun with the 'get about". It is a device that is like a scooter for one leg. I am able to maneuver and steer my way around the house, and/or store with little to no assistance. My girl just has to be the one pushing the shopping cart!

With all of this time to think, and wait for the next step, it seemed to be time to share the full extent of what I have been through with you. I will continue to crack the jokes and find the humor because laughter is the best medicine. Also, I refuse to allow the cancer to define who I am. It is not who I am. While it took more from me than most people realize, it will never define who I am. Only I can give it that power, and that is one power that I refuse to give it . . . no matter how aggressive it may have been, or may still be in the future.

Meanwhile, it is time to go to the store and start preparing for our celebration tonight.

55
The Waiting Game

This is perhaps the hardest time. It is the time of 'wait and see'. I still have two weeks to go before I have my scans and another week after that before I go and get the results. Chemo and radiation have been completed, surgery over months ago, and now we wait and wonder.

I find myself pondering the great truths of the world as I sit in my waiting time. One of the questions that most plagues my mind is one that is unusual for a teacher of English . . . it is a question of terminology.

I know many of the various patterns defining the difference between a plural and a singular word form. I am not sure how to address terms that cover items created by a set that is no longer a set, but a singular entity. Namely, I find myself looking down when I dress in my typical summer wardrobe (a tank top and shorts) and I notice how things don't hang the same. Using the prosthesis does not completely recreate all of a woman's curves. At times like this, I wonder . . . if you only have half of your cleavage, does that mean you just have a cleave?

I am quite certain that it is more noticeable to me than to anyone else in the world . . . after all, I had that other breast as part of my body for the better part of 40 years, so it is only normal that I am noticing its absence. More than missing the actual breast tissue though, I find myself missing other things . . . like the ½ of the cleavage that I don't know what to call. I also am unsure what the proper term for the hole that was left under my arm is supposed to be called. I feel certain that there is a proper name for it. Modified radical mastectomies have been around for a while after all.

Not being something new and different, I know that there must be a term for that area where they removed the lymph nodes and left a hole that cleaves to the rib bones, but I have never been told the term, so I just don't know what to call it. (Perhaps it qualifies as 'underarm cleavage'. . . Thus eliminating the need to change the term 'cleavage' . . . just the location . . .)

I'm sure that these imponderables don't really matter to the majority of polite society. After all, I would not want to show up at a social event and in polite company begin discussing the finer points of the breast amputation process. Some folks might find it just a touch "off-putting". (I have found that the main reason so many people don't talk about these things is that they are still in the category of 'private'. . . like pregnancy used to be. They just are not nearly as pleasant.)

The broken ankle has been both a literal and a figurative pain. I am finally beginning to feel more energetic and have been craving going walking as I did until the treatments made it impossible for me to have the stamina to go. I have not even been able to participate in the water aerobics for the past two months. I was enjoying them so much before the radiation burns got so bad. Now that they are close to healing, I can't participate because, while it would be no problem getting into the pool, climbing out on that ladder would be very difficult with a broken ankle. (I am probably about two weeks away from being able to do that too. Maybe I am just getting impatient.) I do feel myself becoming stronger with every day that passes. My ankle is growing new bone, and the skin over my scar is almost healed. With the leftovers from the burns, I have tremendous scaring. The nicest thing about having this magnitude of scars is, even in a swimsuit, the only people besides me, (and a cast of thousands of medical personnel) Bruce and Zoe are the only ones that will see them. They don't seem to mind.

Hopefully, after we receive the results of the scans we will be able to let the wonderfully supportive administration at the school where I teach know what to expect this year. I know that at the very least I will have scans every four months. I may have (and am hoping to have) reconstructive surgery that will take some additional healing time. Meanwhile, each day I feel a little bit stronger than the day before.

Whatever the results, I hope I remember to ask my medical team what the proper terms are for ½ a cleavage and a hole under the arm.

56
CAT Scans and Plastic Surgeons

There has never in my life been a test that I wanted to ace so badly. The test in question was the follow up to my chemo and radiation . . . my first CAT scan since the cancer treatment.

Poor Zoe had to get up early and accompany me to Odessa for the CAT scans. We left here right at 7:30 am to make it to my 9:30 am appointment. Since I was required to be fasting for the scans, I had Zoe make herself breakfast before we left with a promise of a nice lunch together later on.

Happily, it was one of those days where things were running smoothly at the Oncology offices.

We arrived and checked in with no problems. Of course, I headed straight for the bathroom since that is always high on my priority list after a long drive. As I was coming out of the restroom, my name was being called to go into the lab for blood tests.

Every time a cancer patient will be seeing the Oncologist, blood is drawn so that the doctor can check for what they call cancer markers. Evidently, when cancer is present in the body, certain protein markers frequently may appear in the blood that indicate that there might be a problem. There are different markers for the different types of cancers. Evidently, it is something within the blood that is either elevated or drops to indicate that the body is trying to combat a problem within. In the case of breast cancer, the hormone levels in hormone positive cancers are indicators, or certain proteins or DNA within triple negative breast cancers. According to the American Cancer Society, this only works with more advanced cancers though . . . not with early stage cancer. I guess I should say "lucky for me" that mine was a Stage III from the start so that they can use the markers to help monitor my recovery.

My fellow patient while in the lab was a lovely lady in a wig who was wondering about when her hair would come back and what to expect. We had a lively conversation about medications and hair growth. (Things with us old folks have livened up since the days when all strangers talked about was the weather!)

After the lab-work was done, I had been told to check back in with the receptionist who immediately sent me to chemo for my port flush. As happens frequently, I had a nurse working with me who was not familiar with what we came to term my "pissy port". (Every 2 months, as long as I continue to have my port in place, I must have it 'flushed' to keep it "happy" . . . or from forming clots and becoming blocked and possibly infected.) I explained to the new person about my port, and she, of course, knew better than I possibly could know how to access it . . . which means that after multiple tries on her part, I gave her the name of a couple of the oncology nurses who had worked with it before and knew how rotten it could be. B was brought in to enjoin the battle, and after multiple tries on her part, the nurses were finally satisfied that it was as good as they were going to get. After a quick phone call to radiology, they left the tubing in and sent me back to the lobby.

Again, in the lobby, I was to report to the receptionist. I did, and this time she gifted me with a cold bottle of "Banana Smoothie Barium Drink". This was to be my breakfast. Yee Haw.

I know that watching me drink that wonderful concoction with tubes hanging out of the top of my shirt, and my hair (now curly on the sides and much too straight on the top . . . something almost like Phyllis Diller's old fright wig . . . but of which I am just happy to have) must have been entertaining, because there were more patients in the waiting room watching me drink and laughing at my efforts to choke it down than there were watching the big screen TV. (It was tuned to CNN and discussing the current political situation, so I can't imagine that many were laughing at that.) Many of them stated that they were grateful that I was the one drinking my breakfast rather than them. Although I offered to share, there were no takers. (I suspect they were afraid they might choke because they were laughing so hard at me!) One or two of the chemo patients were even holding their sides and sliding down in their chairs as they laughed. At least my predicament brought some folks joy.

After finishing off the 'smoothie' in record time and spending the next five minutes trying to remove all traces of it from my tongue with my teeth, (I may have resembled a cat trying to hack out a hairball) things finally settled down to the routine . . . more or less. Zoe had her Kindle and I had my cell phone. I had just finished posting on Facebook and told Zoe I was going to go to the restroom again when my name was called and I was finally facing the test.

It is only fair to tell you at this point that I was beginning to get something of a headache from no coffee and a poor night's rest. You see, I spent a very restless night . . . I actually cried myself to sleep for the first time in a long time because I so badly want to pass these tests and there is no way to exert control over your own traitorous body to be sure that the results are what you so desperately want them to be. So, I had alternated crying with prayer to make it through to this point.

This time I was working with a lady from the radiology department whom I had never met. She, like most of the others, was on the petite side, with short, dark hair curled under and framing her face. Her most pleasant accessory was her beautiful, reassuring smile, and she put me instantly at ease. After doing a quick assessment of the mastectomy tank top and my tie top pants, she decided that I had no metal that might interfere with the scans and I did NOT have to change into one of the overly ventilated gowns. I was allowed to just lie down on the machine's bed. She then gifted me with a wonderfully warmed sheet which was a God-send in that overly air-conditioned room.

Like dress rehearsal night before the big performance, she sent me through the tubing a couple of times so that I could practice holding my breath on command of the machine. Unfortunately, the machine in practice mode does not require that you hold your breath as long as during the real deal.

Three trips through in practice mode and then she came back in and had the machine inject the contrast through the tubing in my port. She stated that as it worked, I might feel some warmth in my body. (What she forgot to tell me was that the warmth would all be centered in my crotch!)

It was now time for the real test, and she sent me into the machine again. The machine told me, once again, to hold my breath. I inhaled deeply and waited . . . and waited . . . and waited . . . My eyes popped open in alarm because the machine was having me hold the breath much longer this time and I was beginning to wonder if, like Hal from 2001 Space Odyssey, the machine had developed a sick sense of humor that would require me to hold my breath until I passed out.

The countdown on the pictograph showing me to hold my breath was down to 13. I had not looked at where it began. It was an exceedingly long 13 seconds.

Finally, I could breathe again, and we were done.

On occasion, when I will be in Odessa for medical reasons, Bruce will have me pick up needed items that are easier to come by in the larger city. Today's assignment was a cat carrier for the kitten so that we could keep her safe while the house was being sprayed for roaches. CVS didn't have any, so I used my cell phone to find a PetSmart. (I often wonder how we managed to get anywhere without cell phones through the first half of my life! I can't leave the house without mine now.)

Never take a nearly 12 year old girl who has a new kitten that she is wild about to PetSmart. She didn't want much . . . just one of everything that they had to offer in the cat aisles . . . and there were 4 aisles and a huge chunk of the side wall all devoted to cats.

I finally managed to steer us out of there with a reminder that if we were going to have lunch before the next doctor that we needed to go. But, that did not occur until after she had loved on every dog on a leash that had come into the store . . . one of them multiple times!

Our next stop was Jason's Deli, where we had our usual soup and salad bar, after which we cruised through a shop or two, killing time before our appointment with the plastic surgeon.

We didn't kill enough time.

I could not remember if my appointment was at 1:15, or 1:30, so I decided that it would be best to get there around 1:00. Sadly for us, the doctor's staff did not return to the office until just prior to our appointment time at 1:15.

There is no real lobby area in the building where the plastic surgeon has his offices. That was not as much of a problem, however, as the fact that the temperature had already reached 103 degrees Fahrenheit outside and the building does not provide any type of air conditioning in the hallways or public access areas. Thus, Zoe and I spent a good 30 minutes standing in the heat with no breeze waiting. It did create a nice transition to the air conditioning when we were allowed into the doctor's lobby, however.

Other than the wait, being the first appointment after lunch is a nice place to be. The service is exceptional. I was escorted back into one of the exam rooms where I barely had time to change into my gown before the doctor arrived.

Did I mention that my doctor looks just like the comedian, Steve Martin?

Once again the doctor went over the risks of the tram flap surgery with me and asked me if I realize that I am "high risk" because of my weight. I told him that I do realize that, and explained the setbacks that I have experienced (such as the broken ankle and before that the radiation burns) in trying to get back to a more reasonable weight. He looked at the scarred tissue where my breast once was, and the nurse winced at the sight of the extreme burn scars over the surgical scars.

The agreement was that he will try. He said that he is a bit 'gun-shy' about doing the surgery on me because the last two he has done on overweight women have had complications crop up. I can understand his feelings . . . I was watching him and thinking about how it will feel to have Steve Martin operating on me. After thinking through all of that, my attitude was "third time is a charm".

July 16 is my son's 20th birthday. It is also the date of my 'remodel'. I like to tell people that on the 20th anniversary of my first C section, I will have my belly turned into a boob. (I don't know why, but it tickles me to see people 'snort' in amusement.)

57
Results

Ladies and Gentlemen . . . the results are in.

It is strange to consider that today is, as Dr. K1 put it, an anniversary of sorts. It was one year ago today that I first went to the doctor with the sudden lump that had appeared in my breast. Seems only fitting that today was the day we got the results from the first CAT scans after completion of the chemotherapy and radiation.

Leading up to getting the results, we have had many nights of tossing and turning and worry. I have done my best to not let my fears carry over to the rest of the family and believe that I have done fairly well with it. (Having neighborhood kids set off fireworks outside our bedroom window in the middle of the night early Wednesday morning didn't help in the sleep arena.) Fortunately, Bruce works in enough of a physical environment and long enough hours that many nights he sleeps well due to pure physical exhaustion. I have not been so lucky since I am still somewhat limited due to the healing ankle.

I received a call from the plastic surgeon's office yesterday. They told me that I have been preapproved by the insurance company for my reconstructive surgery, and that I needed to pick up some papers and go to the hospital to do my preadmission work up so that all we need to do on the 16th is to show up. Since my appointment to receive the results from the CAT scan was not scheduled until 11am, we decided to get the paperwork ball rolling first.

Because it is 95 miles to the doctors' offices, we left home about 7:30 am and headed to Odessa. The drive over was uneventful, which, of course, is always the best kind of trip. Bruce took the day off so that he could drive us and be there to hear for himself what Dr. K1 had to say. (He was also support whether the report from the CAT was good or bad.) Bruce drove. Zoe and I each had our Kindles and were reading through the trip. (I am currently reading the second book in the Fifty Shades of Gray trilogy. All I can say is "Oh, my!")

We parked in the parking building and went across to Dr. F's office (he is the one who looks just like Steve Martin.) and were in and out with no problems. They even gave us a map to get to the building where we needed to pre-register me for the pending bodywork. (As I recently told a friend, you might say that I am heading into the shop for some body work on my chassis.)

By 9:15, we were in the correct building and waiting in line to complete the pre-registration for the pending surgery. There was one very small boy who was screaming almost non-stop. His mother was frustrated and would literally drag him from point to point in the waiting room by holding his hand in such a way as to apply pressure to the back of his hand with her thumb, pushing hard between the bones of his hand. It looked painful and I could not blame him for screaming. He was only about 2 years old and she became frustrated when she tried to teach him to play Angry Birds on her cell phone and he was not successful in his efforts. It was sad to watch.

We only had about a 10 minute wait until my name was called and I was able to take care of the paperwork. We concluded that business quickly, and then travelled to the lab for all of the required blood work, EKG, and x-rays. I headed to the back when my name was called this time, leaving Bruce and Zoe in the waiting room with the TV.

The dreaded scales came first. (I really dislike weighing . . . can't believe that I am so heavy!) That was quickly followed by the lab work. I was asked if I mind having a student in the room and I replied that the more the merrier. I pointed out to her that I wear a medical alert bracelet to keep anyone from taking blood pressure or using needles on my left side. Apparently, she was VERY new . . . and they assigned her to do my blood draw. (I suspect that I may have been her very first *ever.*) I asked her to be smooth, and she thought that meant to go very s-l-o-w-l-y with the needle insertion. I don't know if you realize it, but when they stick you slowly, it hurts. When she got done, she was unable to get any blood because she had gone through and through. Her supervisory nurse pulled the needle back into the vein and managed to let the young student draw the remaining needed vials.

Next came the EKG. The supervising nurse was a bit flustered from the blood draw, and tried to explain what she was doing to me to the trainee as she applied the sticky connectors. Realizing that I was wearing a shirt with a prosthesis in it, she decided to not have me remove my shirt. (What little she saw of my scars seemed to make her VERY uncomfortable.) Unfortunately, she was not paying enough attention to what she was doing and was unable to get a reading on the machine after hooking up the leads. She pulled up two leads and readjusted them. That didn't work, so she moved another three of the sticky connections (and some of my skin each time) and my heart still did not register. Finally, she retraced her steps and discovered that she had not connected the final lead to my right upper arm. Once connected, the machine was able to take the EKG readings. She had to try twice to get it to print, but she finally succeeded. (I believe that she was quite flustered by then, because she proceeded to RIP the lead lines off of me. I have not yet checked, but I am certain that I will find holes in my skin where the tape was ripped off!)

Next, I was taken to wait for x-rays of my chest. When I came into the room, I was asked to change into a 'breezy gown'. While the ladies did not see my scars on the surface, I know they saw the internal radiation damage by their verbal wincing when they took the x-rays.

Finally, I was sent back to the waiting room where I was told to wait to receive instructions from "the prep nurse".

We waited. We waited. We waited and waited. Finally, at 10:52, knowing that we had an 11am appointment with Dr. K1 to get the results of the CAT scans, I approached the docent (the volunteers who help things in the hospital to run smoothly) who was manning the desk. He told me that there was nothing he could do about it, and I would just need to wait. Before I could get really angry at his lack of assistance, one of the lab ladies came out to call a different patient. I explained the situation to her and she took my phone number down to give to the nurse. (After finishing at the oncology office, we went back and were told that the nurse will probably not call me until the Friday before the surgery . . . Hey! That will be on

Friday the 13th!)

The appointment we have been losing sleep over was finally upon us. Fortunately, it was just 2 blocks over from where we were to where we needed to be to receive the big results.

After meeting with Dr. K1, we have decided that we will have to resign ourselves to the fact that we will never hear "You are cured", or that "It is over" . . . or probably even never hear "You are in remission". There are just too many missing parts in my body, and too much scar tissue from the missing parts. I am anxious to start losing the weight that they put on me with the chemo and radiation diets though. I feel like I will feel much better if I can finally get that to start happening. Dr. K1 assures us that I "appear" to be fine at this time. He stressed that he feels that the 'abnormalities' that were seen in the CAT scan were the result of the radiation changes. I need a follow up in 4 months. At that time, he has ordered another CAT scan and a fresh mammogram the month before the visit.

At any rate, the summary report from the CAT scan reads as follows:

IMPRESSION:

1. No definite evidence of intra-abdominal metastatic disease although the underlying fatty infiltration of the liver significantly limits evaluation for hepatic metastasis, consider ultrasound for further evaluation.
2. Mass like area lower pole left kidney likely related to adjacent scarring rather than a true renal mass, comparison to prior studies or attention on follow-up.
3. Sclerosis mid left sternum is indeterminate.

Not the most positive report I have ever received, but maybe it will make us sleep better. Right now, the prognosis is to wait and see yet again.

58
Pre-Reconstruction Musings

I have been researching again.

In preparation for my coming remodeling surgery on Monday, I decided to look up the Tram Flap reconstruction and the projected recovery times. I started with the images and finished up by reading blogs of other women who have had the surgery done and how it affected them. I even went to the extent of emailing to one of them and received a reply from her within the hour!

In beginning the research, I had many unusual questions . . . some of which would be considered by some as "inappropriate". (It seems to me like I frequently do that "inappropriate" thing.)

My first question came up the other day when I was musing about the newest pending changes in my body. I remembered a conversation that I had with my dear friend Vera' when she was going through her cancer fight. She had received the Latissimus Dorci rebuild at the time of her mastectomy. (In other words, they used her back muscles to build her new breast.) She told me one time that when her husband became amorous and began to rub, it felt to her like she was receiving a back rub. That got me to thinking (dangerous, I know), since I am being rebuilt using my belly, will mine have the sensations of the belly.

Deciding to take advantage of the quick shot at humor, I called to my daughter, "Hey, Zoe. I was just thinking about my procedure and wondering . . . since they are making my new breast from my belly . . . if I get a bellyache, will my new boob hurt?"

Ever the literal child, Zoe responded, "No, Momma. When you get a bellyache, it is actually discomfort arising in your stomach or intestines. Since neither of those will be moved, it is highly unlikely that you will have a bellyache in your boob."

She knows how to kill a joke . . . and she is only 11 and speaks so formally!

Today's research showed that to a great extent, she was right. It told me that for most women, so many nerves are cut in the re-arranging process that there is usually little to no sensation in the reconstructed breast. Those who do have sensation tend to report numbness and not much else.

With that piece of information firmly established and verified by sources more reliable than Wikipedia, I was left with only one other question that has been nagging at me. No matter how much I researched, I was unable to find any reference that would answer my other nagging question.

In discussions with friends, we have joked a bit about it, but no one has been forthcoming with the answer.

I have always tended to be a somewhat hairy woman. One of the places that I have had hair the majority of my life is the line of hair that runs from under my bellybutton down.

Knowing that my new breast skin will be the skin transferred from under my bellybutton to my breast--I wonder if I will, after things settle in, need to shave my new breast.

One of my friends from work says that this dilemma gives a whole new meaning to putting hair on your chest.

59
After the Body Shop

I now know how the bottom of the glass feels (if the bottom of the glass could feel) when someone uses the straw to slurp the last few drops of fluid.

This has been the most interesting week of my yearlong cancer ordeal. I have travelled many new roads, most of which I would not wish on my worst enemy, and met many wonderful people who would never have come into my life had the cancer not made an appearance.

What I have discovered on this journey is that the cancer survivors tend to be very giving, loving people with a tremendous capacity to care and offer comfort to others who are likewise afflicted. It has been a humbling experience to now realize that I must count myself among their numbers. I have made new friends from all around the world in the cancer groups that I have joined, and I no longer hesitate to email a stranger who has placed their story, or some part of their journey online for the world to see and possibly be helped by it. While it is a very personal journey, and highly emotional, physically draining, and hell on the budget, those who have been there remain there for the next one in line to receive that diagnosis. Having made it thus far, the little things are not nearly as worrisome as they were before the doctor spoke those dreaded words. Life has taken on a deeper, more meaningful existence than was readily obtainable before. B.C . . . Before Cancer.

I now find myself in another semantics dilemma after this week's surgery. What do I call the 'hanger on'? Technically, she is no longer a

Cyclops because she now has company and is no longer alone. (I find myself looking forward to my reduction and lift though. It is hard to wake up in the morning, look in the mirror while I dress, and not die laughing at the differences between my new, perky belly-boob and the other who appears to be racing at warp speed for my knee . . . and right now it hurts when I laugh!) I suppose that I will go with a suggestion made by my niece and start to call her the "Sole Survivor". The new one, of course, is destined to be the "Belly-Boob".

Before we got to this point, though, last Monday we made another trip to Odessa. This time we were heading for the first of the rebuild procedures. We were on our way to another surgery, but it was worth it because I was finally going to get my TRAM Flap procedure done.

In the prep room, Dr. F tried his best to prepare us for the worst case scenarios. He told Bruce to let the rest of the family (who were waiting in the waiting room downstairs) know that he expected the surgery to take a minimum of five hours. As we headed for the OR, Bruce gave me one more kiss for luck as we stopped at the restroom to allow me one more trip to empty my bladder, and then we were off.

Since I prefer my OR team to be relaxed, I was glad when we came through the doors and classic rock was playing as they were getting things ready to go. I grinned and called out, "Let's get this party started!"

We transferred me onto the operating table (which was the first one that I have been on that didn't feel like parts of me would be on the floor before we were done), where Dr. F had me sit up so that he could draw the dotted lines on me like he was about to shape some paper dolls. He then had me lie down and as I put my arms out (dizzy spinning circle style) and the staff began to strap down my legs, I called out, "Hey . . . wait a minute . . . what kind of a party did you say this was?" (I really shouldn't have read the "50 Shades of Grey" trilogy last week!)

The anesthesiologist told me that he was giving me a shot to help me relax, and true to form, I was out until I woke up in recovery.

I was later told that, much to Dr. F's surprise, my surgery went without any problems and was over in four hours. I was installed in my room right at five hours after Bruce and I parted ways for the surgery to begin. When I came to, the nurse who was monitoring me in the recovery room asked me how I felt and I asked her if anyone had gotten the license plate number of the truck that hit me. She apologized and stated that she didn't realize that was what had happened to me. I quickly explained what I had just had done and that I was making a joke. (She wasn't even blonde!)

Sometimes we never learn. I tried the same quip with another medical person on the way to my hospital room and received the same result. I really need to remember that (unlike my wonderful step-sons and their wives) most medical people seem to have had their sense of humor removed. (Maybe it is the first procedure they practice on one another . . .)

With this type of surgery, the first concern is that the new boob that was made from the belly might not latch on. It is checked frequently for temperature and color. By the time that 48 hours had passed, Dr. F quipped, "I think we got away with it!" There was color response when it is touched, and another sign was that the hair they had shaved from my belly at the start of the procedure was beginning to regrow in its relocated spot.

The answer about hair growth is that yes, I will need to shave, wax, or have the hair removed by laser during the follow-up procedures. In short, I have a well-established 5 o'clock shadow on my new belly boob. (I just love giving the world more to laugh with me about! Fortunately, Bruce loves me . . . hairier chest than him and all!)

This time, I had three of the suction bulbs starting out. I managed to have the top one removed before we left the hospital on Thursday. (Yes, I beat that timeline too!) That leaves me with the two that are located down south where my body so graciously and unknowingly grew and donated my new booby. They are numbered and number 2 seems to be on a mission to suck out as much fluid from my body as possible. This is how I know how it feels to be the bottom of the glass.

I had been experiencing what (to me at least) was rather serious leakage issues. Dr. F told me to just use my panties to hold on the bandages because of my tape issues. (Some of the blisters from the tape that was on my belly are HUGE! I have one that clocks in larger than a quarter and stands ½ an inch high. I dread when it finally pops.)

After traveling to the pharmacy with my parents this morning to get my pain medication prescription filled, I decided that I needed to do something. The bulbs did not appear to be pulling out the fluid, but it was backing up strongly onto my panties and shorts. I headed for the bathroom to try and find a solution.

Following Dr. F's advice, I had used the panties to hold on the bandages (which were now soaked) and safety pins to attach the bulbs to the waistband of my shorts. I decided to think in terms of gravity and try a different track.

Ditching the now soaked panties, I threw away the sopping bandages and threaded the suction bulbs through the legs of my shorts, where I pinned them to the hem…one to each leg. Using fresh gauze, I wrapped the tubing thoroughly and by holding it when I walked back into the den, I was able to keep them inside my shorts until I reached my recliner. (Always one to see myself from the view of a fly on the wall, I decided that I did not look any less dignified than the 'wanna-bes' who hold their waistband at their crotch . . . small comfort . . . but I must be 'styling'.)

With the new changes in place, within 30 minutes, I had suctioned out a full five ounces with tube 2. I emptied it and it began to immediately refill before I even left the bathroom! But, since Baby's britches are dry finally, she doesn't care how stupid she looks walking back and forth down the hall! Besides, it is only temporary.

I will go in for my first post-surgical checkup on Tuesday. I will let you know how things go after that.

60
Surgeries and Wound Vac

Well, the cancer didn't manage to kill me, but the rebuild tried to.

On July 16, the 20th anniversary of my first C-Section, I was admitted into the hospital and Dr. F. performed a TRAM Flap surgery on me. The TRAM Flap is a very interesting surgery. It uses the main stomach muscle (the 'sit-up' muscle) for the blood supply. It is left attached to the belly which is detached and moved through a created pocket between the outer skin and the ribcage and used to create a replacement breast for the one that was lost through the mastectomy. Given the nature of the changes, for a while, I referred to the new breast as my 'belly-boob'. This only lasted until I got home on July 19. My daughter's cat climbed onto my lap and proceeded to hiss and growl at the new breast. It brought to mind images of Frankenstein from the old black and white movie, and was transformed forever in my mind to "Franken-Boob".

Dr. F had warned me that I would experience extreme fatigue and that it would take from six months to a year to feel like myself again. I was prepared for that. What I was unprepared for was the 'wasting away' that began to set in shortly after I returned home.

One of the bonus side effects from the TRAM Flap is that on a select number of us, our system feels and reacts as if it has had a bariatric surgery in addition to everything else. I was delighted to find my over-sized self in this elite group that would end up losing weight after the surgery. I was not delighted as things proceeded to become rather 'touch and go' for my body. I made it to the first post op check fine. By the second week after the surgery, however, I had basically become bed ridden. I was running a constant low-grade fever. I was force feeding myself, and dropping 3-4.5 lbs per day. I had developed what is best described as a 'vomit-cough' that was so horrible sounding that my daughter would break down in tears every time I coughed. It was rather scary. The day that I went for my second post op check, Dr. F had me admitted to the hospital. Since I suspected that things were getting bad enough to die, I didn't quibble about the quick admission.

Bruce was marvelous, as were my parents. He had me text him a list of things I would need for my hospital stay, and made the double long trip home before coming to see us (my daughter was with me) in the hospital. My parents made arrangements and headed down immediately to watch over Zoe while I was in the hospital.

All of the lab work that was done came back showing a woman in perfect health. I didn't have an elevated white count. My lung x-rays were perfect. I did show an elevation in my blood sugar, but that did not account for the 'vomit-cough', nor the low-grade fever.

I was admitted on Tuesday. By Thursday, August 1 . . . the 1st anniversary of my mastectomy . . . the decision was made to operate and see what was happening in Franken-Boob. (Swabs that were taken from some of the 'jucier' places on Franken-Boob showed bacterial growths in spite of the fact that I did not have an elevated white count.)

Because I was a late addition to the surgical schedule, I was the last surgery of the day on Thursday. I was finally moved into the operating room about 2pm where I went gratefully to sleep and away from all my discomforts.

It is a mark of how bad things were that by the next morning, in spite of the now open tunnel in my chest, I felt remarkably better. Franken-Boob had developed two abscesses . . . one on the side of my sternum, and the other under my arm . . . which Dr. F removed. To monitor healing and prevent development of additional abscesses, the wound was left packed with very wet gauze (which leaked all over my ventilated gown, sheets, and anything I touched) and covered with the super thick belly bandages that are normally reserved for belly wounds. (Given the nature of Franken-Boob's existence, I thought the belly bandages were very appropriately appropriated to the use.)

Wrapped this way, Dr. F brought in two sets of specialists to work with me. To address the blood sugar issues, he had me moved to a diabetic diet, and had my sugars monitored by one of the 'hospitalists'. (A hospitalist is a doctor who works for the hospital but does not have his/her own private practice.) For the dressing of the wounds in my chest, Dr. F brought in the highly specialized Wound Care division of the medical facility. They handled my wound dressing changes on Friday and Saturday. One of my awesome nurses (all of whom I left loving dearly) did the changes on Sunday.

Given the length of my stay and the uncertainty of everything, my parents took my girl back home with them so that they could take care of their personal business. This allowed my husband (who was out of leave time because he used it all on me for my chemo) to continue working. (Sadly, bills still need to be paid and money needs to come in even though a family member is in the hospital.)

Monday, August 6, I went into surgery again. Again, I was the last on the queue, but this time, it was after 5pm before they got me into the operating room. As I was wheeled into the O.R., Dr. F thanked me for "having the patience of Job". Again, the necrotic tissues were removed. This time, however, the two wounds became one. The best description that I can come up with is when we were kids and it would (on those rare occasions) snow. We would mound the snow into a hill and try to dig a tunnel through. This is what Franken-Boob now resembled.

Backing up the story for a minute . . . the blood sugar had become a constant issue. I even did battle with the hospital dietician who insisted that the hospital diabetic diet was a true diabetic diet. The longer I was on it, the higher my blood sugar went. Every diabetic meal was accompanied by potatoes, white bread or biscuits, and pie or cake. Breakfast would be eggs with pancakes, French toast, white toast, or blueberry muffins. They even substituted a fruit cup for my bacon one morning!

The dietician tried to tell me that the potatoes were the same carb count as a package of crackers. Their meals were based on 'units'. Each food that is a high carb food was given one unit and they assigned 5-6 units to each meal (which left their diet extremely high carb!) Since returning home and eating the way I normally do, my blood sugars have returned to normal, only going up again when I go in to wound care and receive their two hour dressing change.

After Monday's surgery, we were left with the question of what to do with the closure of Franken-Boob. Dr. F and Wound Care decided that a wound vac was the perfect solution.

The wound vac consists of a vacuum unit attached to the outside of the wound. The inside of the wound is packed with colorful sponges; black, white, red, blue, and purple, which assist in helping the wound to heal from the inside out. After the sponges are pieced together inside, the outside is covered with clear tape that will allow the wound to seal. A suction pump is applied through the outer clear bandages and it proceeds to suck out all air and any draining fluids. (Supposedly, it will allow my tunnel to seal up naturally ten times faster than any other method of trying to heal such a large wound.)

When the wound vac was first applied, I was given a very large, bulky, heavy machine to carry. It had a battery life of one hour and I was tethered by extension cords. When the first bandaging change took place on Friday, the large pack was replaced with a small, highly portable pack that slings over my shoulder. It has a battery life in the 8-10 hour range. While the machine is labeled as a "VacUlta", we are constantly glancing at the name and saying and thinking "Vacula". (Seems fitting that "Vacula" would be the healing source of "Franken-Boob".)

My daughter, Zoe, was unable to look at Franken-Boob before the abscess. Now, she thinks it is really cool to watch (after the sponges are changed) when the machine is first turned on. I, on the other hand, feel something like one of those vacuum storage bags that you suck the air out of and then stuff under the bed. I am glad that we have a waterbed and I don't fit underneath it. I am a bit afraid someone might stuff me under there!

Long term, I will have home health care come 2 days a week to change my sponges, and I will travel to Odessa once per week for Wound Care to monitor my healing progress. It seems like I can never be the person who does things the easy way.

61
The Saga Continues After the Wound Vac

And the healing process continues.

For one month, I wore the wound vac. It was always amazing to see the tremendous progress each time that the bandages were changed. When the sponges were removed, there was visible growth to the internal tissues that are needed to fill in under where the skin grafts will be.

The most amusing day during the time with the wound vac was the day that I noticed one of my sophomore boys staring, mesmerized by the fluids moving through the tubing on the wound vac. Without taking his eyes from the tubes, he asked me if it was blood moving through the tubes. I responded that it was. He then became really quiet and thoughtful before looking up at me in genuine concern and asking, "Is it yours?"

Unfortunately, a different home health agency than the one that was used the first time was hired to assist me with this stage of the treatment and they had been somewhat reluctant to meet my schedule. Everything was fine until school resumed and I went back to work. At that point, they were rather vocal about not wanting to come to my house for the hour long sponge and bandage changes at 4 p.m. They first wanted me to take off work so that they would not have to work after 4:00. Next, they wanted to prove to me that I could have the change done during my 47 minute lunch break. In an effort to prove this, the nurse in charge of the paperwork showed up to do the change and ripped the sponges out of the wound without loosening them first. I bawled like a baby.

Trying to make herself feel better about making me cry (and hurting me badly enough that I spent the next 24 hours wishing I had morphine available) she looked at me and said, "I bet you have cried lots of times during this, haven't you!?"

My response was a bit more direct than it would have been in the past. I replied, "No, Ma'am. I did not cry with the cancer. I did not cry with the mastectomy. I did not cry with chemo or radiation even when the burns went nearly to the bone. You, Ma'am, are the only person throughout this whole ordeal who has managed to make me cry."

She followed up by using extra drape (the clear tape that is used to seal in the sponges) without using the tape prep on my skin beforehand. I reminded her that I have some serious issues with tape and she proceeded to tell me that it would be fine because she had done it on the good skin, not skin that was radiated and therefore more susceptible to tearing. (The tape burned my 'good skin' to the point of blisters that have now turned to scars. What it didn't burn had a hives-like rash when the Wound Care center next saw me. They were not pleased.)

On August 27, the home health agency took fluid samples from the wound to send to the lab because of the odor that I kept complaining about that was coming from the wound. When I went to the Wound Care Center for treatment on September 7, the smell was much worse, and they decided that they should take some samples and send them to the lab. I asked what the results had been from the tests done by the home health agency. They had never received the results, nor did they even know that samples had been taken.

After immediately calling the home health agency and requesting the results to be sent, the wound care center told me that the lab report which was faxed over showed a bacterial infection and even recommended specific antibiotics to be used to treat it. Unfortunately, in the ensuing 12 days, the infection had increased from where it was when the original reports were made and become much more pronounced.

While the wound vac had helped to slow the progression of it, the bacterial infection was increasing. The decision was made to change me to a 'wet dressing' with changes of the bandages twice a day while I was on the antibiotics. This also would allow my skin a chance to heal since I was able to hold the bandages in place with my post-surgical bra rather than continuing the use of tape or drape (both of which had left my skin with another hives-like rash).

As I sit here writing this, I am wondering if I will be doing my own bandage changes from now on. I have the new orders for the local home health agency, yet when the head nurse brought bandages by on Friday night (after I called a second time to get the materials and she still had not arrived by 9:30 pm), she rushed in and out without collecting the orders. She knows that they are supposed to change the bandages once per day, and I am to change them once per day, but she does not want to come here to do it.

At least I know that I will get to see my surgeon again on Tuesday. Hopefully, the infection will be better by then, and we can look toward scheduling my last surgery.

62
More Waiting

Everything in life is a process. I frequently must remind myself of this fact, and work at remaining patient and trusting in God to get me through this process. However, I must confess that I am tired of the whole thing. Cancer and cancer recovery just take too long and impatience for it to be resolved kicks in with alarming regularity. I think that this is why the waiting that is going on right now drives me nuts. I miss the spontaneity that we once had as a family that allowed us to just pick up and go on the weekends when and where we wanted. Now, we are so aware of the need to save money (cancer is not cheap) that if we did go anywhere there is not much that I could do. Being restricted to lifting no more than 8 lbs. is also very limiting, and knowing that I have the open wounds on my chest puts a damper on most anything even slightly physical.

While we are waiting and hoping for the desired end to this process, I find myself each day meeting someone who is something of a stranger to me. When I look in the mirror, I don't look like the same person that I was for 48 years . . . chemo changed that. And my personality has also grown in ways that sometimes surprise me.

I once described myself to my new boss as being so type B that I am often mistaken for dead. One of the biggest changes in my personality seems to be that those who are mistaking me for dead and acting on it find out rather abruptly that I am not dead, and my BS tolerance (as I stated in my last notes) is virtually non-existent anymore. (I can't help but come home and laugh privately at the expressions on faces of people who have run over me in the past when they find that I am no longer in doormat mode!) I have no need to strike back because I really believe that the world is round for a reason. Whatever you throw out there at others will eventually come back around and "Gibbs slap" you in the back of the head!

The biggest problem with all of this waiting time is that there is just too much time to think. I manage to keep the demons at bay most of the time by planning and preparing for the next step in the fight, but right now I am in limbo . . . not knowing if I need to keep fighting, or if the fight has been won, so I keep on running the race and wondering where the finish line might be hiding.

My other "demon-halting" hobby is to look long and hard at myself and my situation and find all of the humor that I can. It is a blessing that there is so much about me to laugh about! (I am supremely grateful that God had such a good sense of humor when putting me together!)

My hair is getting longer. (I am delighted that I have the hair!) Having never before had naturally curly hair, I am never sure what to do with it, so most of the time I let it grow wild. I did notice and point out to my students a couple of days ago, however, that I am very glad it is not red. If it were, in its current style, I would begin to resemble Ronald McDonald! (The day after I made this observation, God took pity on me and my hair finally began to calm down and start to lie down!)

I am very pleased to say that the weight loss has continued. I am down 31 lbs. from when I came home in July from the rebuild. This puts me only 12 lbs. to my pre-chemo weight. (Do you realize that at 31lbs down, I have lost an average sized toddler? It's a good thing too, because I am getting too old to keep up with a toddler!)

Yet, the waiting continues. Currently, I am waiting for my next surgery to be scheduled. When I met with the doctor week before last, we agreed to do a two-for-one. He will do the reduction on the Cyclops and a lift to make it match Franken-boob, and he will use the extra materials from the Cyclops to fill-in and graft on Franken-boob. He will also remove my chemo port while he is at it. All we are waiting on is for the pre-authorization from the insurance company. They are taking their time. (They keep sending me letters wanting me to list everyone in the household and what insurance they have because they really want me to have another insurance that could help them with these bills!)

I am also rapidly approaching my next set of tests. My mammogram is scheduled for the first week in October. (Happily, I will only need to be tortured on the side of the Cyclops! Franken-boob, while posing as a breast is still in origin my belly, and mammograms are not performed on bellies.) I wonder if the insurance company will only need to pay half-price since the mammogram will only cover one side . . . Another plus is that since this mammogram is not diagnostic, the insurance should cover it completely! (I was shocked last year when I received the bill for my mammogram. It seems that while it is exactly the same test performed whether as an annual screening, or a diagnostic due to potential cancer, the insurance company will only include it as an annual screening if there is not a suspicion of cancer present beforehand.)

In November, I will have my next CAT scan and get the results from both tests. I am hoping and praying that with this next CAT scan the doctor will, after doing his comparisons to the last set, say that all is looking good and move me to the 6 month intervals from the 4 month that I am currently on. That, more than anything, will make me feel like a survivor more than a patient.

All things considered, I have a confession. The more I get to know the 'changed' me, the better I like and respect the me I am becoming. I have talked with you off and on about balance. That was the physical aspects. Even though physically my balance is still off a bit, I think that my experiences have improved my balance in areas that really count . . . like my lowered tolerance for doormat treatment. In many ways, I am better able to judge when to turn the other cheek and when to throw up a shield and say, "Enough. I am worth more than that. I will not accept you mistreating me, or anyone else for that matter, so that you can feel better about yourself. I suggest you find a different victim if you feel you must belittle someone. I do suggest, however, that you don't do it around me. I will not tolerate that type of behavior in my presence and will go to whatever means are necessary to stop it." (I have found that I am still quicker to reject the BS treatment when I witness it than when I experience it, but I am improving!)

In many ways, I feel like that old commercial from the '70's said, "You're not getting older. You're getting better."

63
Post Cancer Mammogram

Unremarkable. That is my new favorite word. Unremarkable.

Last Thursday was a really busy day. I started the day at by going to Odessa to have my mammogram. The lady who scheduled the appointment for me at the Oncologist office told me that while listed as a 'diagnostic' procedure, I would simply have my mammogram unless they saw something questionable. If they saw a potential problem, then they would perform an ultrasound on the breast as well.

After having the Cyclops squashed and maneuvered in ways that one should only use on Silly Putty or Play Dough, the technician took me back to the dressing room and told me that I would need to wait for my ultrasound.

I tried to read for a bit since I brought my Kindle with me. The information on the door was most informative since I found myself unable to concentrate on my historical fiction while pacing the 3x3 room. (It's hard to pace a 3x3 room, by the way.)

One of the notices on the door stated that women who have dense breast tissue might need to seek alternative means of checking for cancer since statistically, dense tissue could easily hide a cancer. I found this interesting since in all of my mammograms prior to my cancer showing up, I had always been told that while my right breast was normal for my age, the left tended to be more dense . . . as are those of younger women. (At the time, we chalked it up to me aging faster on the right side than the left.)

The technician stuck her head in the door and told me that it was our turn in the ultrasound room.

Unlike Franken-boob's predecessor, the Cyclops forced me to angle myself toward the wall where I was unable to look at the screen and see for myself what they were seeing. This was somewhat stressful for me. Since I was now having an ultrasound, I really needed to be seeing what they were looking at. Sadly, it was not to be.

The technician took her photos and wiped me down. (For these procedures, they always slather you in what feels like high grade hair gel). She then started talking about me getting dressed and waiting to get my results in the mail. With the tears in my eyes that I was trying to banish to my toenails, I asked the technician if anything showed up in the tests. I explained to her that I had been told that they would only do the ultrasound if something questionable was found. She replied that she would ask the doctor if the doctor would tell me her findings. If the lady doc wanted to, she would come in and tell me, but because she was only the technician, as a technician, she could tell me nothing.

And so, I waited.

The doctor who came in when the technician returned was the same one as last year. The primary difference was that somewhere between last year and this year, she seemed to find her sense of humor. (Remember that I wrote to you last year about how she lambasted me for playing a joke on her technician . . . and for having a sense of humor. Last year, she was so dry that she made the character of 'Bones' seem like a comedian!)

The doc smiled at me and stated that my mammogram and ultrasound were totally 'unremarkable'.

I, through my deep sigh of relief, stated that I now had a new favorite word . . . 'unremarkable'.

She laughed and said, "I finally figured it out. Don't ever quit your day job."

My response was, "Okay . . . figured what out?"

"You," she replied, "are a stand-up comedian for your day job."

"In some ways, you are correct. I teach high school."

We went on this way for a few minutes, each laughing, and ended with a "see you next year" (which is another phrase that sounded like music to my ears!)

After leaving there, I walked over to the Oncology clinic. My port has been 'unhappy' lately. The idea was that I could go in and they would 'flush' my port with heparin and break up whatever clots were forming there. One of my favorite chemo nurses jumped on the job and tried to help out. (Ports are supposed to be 'flushed' every 4 weeks. Mine had not been since the end of June, because the hospital had refused to access it when I was there and I honestly had not thought about it when I wasn't there.) On Tuesday night, I had awakened in the middle of the night with a sharp pain that extended through my shoulder and up my neck. I instantly knew that my port was blocked . . . probably with a clot.

Try as she might, my nurse was unable to either draw blood, nor to get any of the heparin into the port. Since I am having it removed next week, I need to just "hang in there" and keep on with my pain pills.

My score for the day now stood at one win, one loss. Next stop was the plastic surgeon's office. In order to have my next surgery, I needed to make a down payment of $400.00 to the office, with a balance of $750.00. (Still don't know where I am going to come up with all that money!)

Since it was Thursday, I knew that the doctor would be in surgery, so I expected to meet with his office manager. However, she was not there, and I met with a very young nurse.

The young nurse successfully managed to relieve me of $400.00, and provide me with the pre-admission packet that I needed to take to pre-admission people for next week's surgery.

Since I don't teach math currently, I decided to count that as two wins with the one loss . . . that put me at three and one for the day.

Next stop was a quick walk to the Wound Care Center. I didn't have a long wait, and I was in. When the doctor asked me how I was doing, I told him that I really need his help. Since my blood pressure was up to 140/90 when it is normally about 120/60, they knew that I was hurting bad. I explained about the blocked port, and they got busy trying to find someone who might be able to remove it. Sadly, while they talked about how wonderful my wounds look, they were unable to find a surgeon who has the proper "hospital permissions" to remove the port. That leaves me with the options of going through an ER and sitting there until they finally find a surgeon who has those permissions, or waiting until next week for the scheduled surgery. I opted to wait it out with the pain pills.

New score for the day was up to four wins and two losses. To me it sounded like it was time for lunch.

Lunch was a wonderful meal at Music City Mall. I had promised my students that I would get some more of the aroma therapy anti-stress lotion for the classroom, so I needed to go to Bath & Body Works to get some. I did that after a quick lunch at Fuddruckers.

After all the fun, (and I didn't even get lost in the mall for a change!) I headed back to the hospital to go through the pre-registration process. It was a short wait . . . only about 45 minutes after I arrived before I was called to go over my medical history and pre-register with the hospital for next week's surgery. The most depressing part was when I filled out the paperwork over lunch and realized that this will be my 15th surgery. Had my wonderful Bruce Batson not been with me through most of them, I wondered if I would have made it. I doubt that I would have. He has been a rock and lent me strength through the years on a regular basis! I continue to hope and pray that this will be the last of the surgeries . . . at least for many years!

I passed my EKG with only a brief pause when the nurse looked at my bandages and had no clue what to do with the leads she needed to attach directly under my left breast (Franken-boob). She saw the bandages and I explained that she was trying to work with my Sunday breast. When she looked at me quizzically, I explained, "It's holy."

She came back from visiting with her supervisor right after that, and set the leads under the bandages. I must give her kudos . . . that was the first time I have had the EKG and not gone home to find surprise leads to remove later on.

That was followed by chest x-rays and a visit with the surgical nurse.

Long story short (I know. I know. Too late.), I will report for surgery next Thursday at 9am. I continue to hope and pray that this is the last one.

Score for the day was five and two. (Wish that our high school football team had a record like that!)

64

Progress

Tonight, words are not adequate to express the feelings of sheer jubilation that are dancing in my soul! This morning, Bruce accompanied me to get the results of this last set of CAT scans, mammogram, ultrasound, and blood work. This has been my life every four months since finishing chemotherapy.

I fully expected to have some issues with this CAT scan. After all, since the one in June, I have had my belly moved up to become a new (albeit hairy) boob to replace the one that I lost to the cancer. Following that, I ended up with two more surgeries to remove the subsequent abscesses, a month wearing a wound vac, and another surgery to finally close up the open wounds and downsize the Cyclops. (At one point, I even accused my plastic surgeon of sponsoring a seeding program rather than just doing the surgery. I told him that he went in to seed the new breast, and then ended up having me grow it myself using the wound vac. He just laughed.)

After the surgeries and holes and moving things around, and healing time, I was hoping to be through for a while. I will continue to have scans periodically, and I still have at least one more surgery to try and fix the deformities that were left from the abscesses and subsequent surgeries to keep me alive. But, it's all good. I am still alive to serve humanity as either a wonderful example or a terrible warning (depending on your perspective). Since my battle scars and current deformities do not seem to bother my wonderful family, they don't bother me.

For years prior to all of this mess, I have maintained a rather indifferent attitude about my appearance. Whenever students would mention a bad hair day, or tell me that I looked tired, my response would be to tell them that it appeared that they had a problem . . . I did not have to look at me, but they were the ones who did! I suppose that this attitude has played a helpful role in my recovery through all of this mess with cancer. If I had been vain, in addition to being somewhat unrealistic about my strengths and weaknesses, I would probably have been much more concerned about each step in this forever process of tearing down through amputation, followed by rebuilding through rearrangement. The only thing that continues to bother me much is how very hairy Franken-boob continues to be.

After having the bandages removed again, (finishing yet another post-surgical round) the first thing I requested was to be allowed to finally shave Franken-boob. (I still can't decide whether it was more funny, or sad, that Dr. F replied, "Please do. That is the hairiest boob I have seen in my career!")

I quickly discovered that shaving Franken-boob did temporarily remove the hair, but the five o'clock shadow was murder on the underside of my arm! (It also tended to catch on my clothing . . . You can't imagine how inconvenient it is to 'beard' the chest area of a sweater . . . especially from the inside!)

Given my options, I ruled out the use of depilatories, and opted instead for privately waxing. Sadly, this means letting the hair grow out again! (It is a strange experience when showering to see that I have more hair on my new breast than I do under my arms . . . not sure how to file that psychological adjustment.) I spend more time in clothing than out, however, so I quietly cover my issues and laugh about them whenever I get the opportunity.

The realization that when Dr. F removed about 4 lbs. of tissue from the Cyclops when he reduced me and only took my DDD down to a D has also been another adjustment. (Unfortunately, Franken-boob came out about a C cup. Cyclops is a D. Buying bras has been interesting. I either go with the stretchy multi-size . . . which I have come to really love . . . or those that have a touch of padding. With these, I add a sock on top of Franken-boob to try and even things out. I have a sort of 'shelf' on top where things healed strangely after the surgeries to remove the abscesses.) I suspect that there will continue to be adjustments as each new surgery happens and things are re-formed to a more normal appearance.

This has been a time of many mental adjustments for me. I finally understand that the periodic CAT Scans and multiple tests will continue for the rest of my life. I was always accustomed to getting sick, fighting it off, and going on like it never happened. I tried to do that with this cancer. It worked as far as keeping me from losing my mind went, but in some ways, it had me in a state of Pollyanna denial. I have recently come to understand how very sick I was and how very close I came to no longer being here. Friends and family recognized it long before I did, and they graciously allowed me to continue in my denial, probably in the hopes that my refusal to accept how it really was would lead to the more favorable outcome that we have now. (You may truly call me "Cleopatra" because I have one year's evidence to prove that I am, in fact, the 'queen of denial'.)

Many wonderful people prayed with me and for me in the hopes that we would see progress with this set of tests. I am happy to report that the very thing we prayed for has come to pass. We prayed that I would be taken off of the schedule of CAT scans every 4 months and placed on a 6 month schedule. The only thing in my current CAT scans that merits watching, Dr. K1 feels, is too insignificant to be a true threat to my health. We will look at it again in May.

Getting to this point is much like having a birthday . . . I feel like today is my 1st birthday. This is when the feelings of success and hope for the future are born and growing as the time passes post treatment. There appears to be a light at the end of the tunnel--and it doesn't feel like a train this time.

Cast of Characters in Life's Drama

Jamie	Me
Bruce	My wonderful hubby
Zoe	My beautiful daughter
Dr. P	My regular physician
Dr. G1	My heart doctor
Dr. G2	My surgeon
Dr. K1	My Oncologist
B	An Oncology Nurse
Dr. A	My Ophthalmologist
Dr. K2	My Radiologist
J	Radiologist's Nurse
Beautiful Buxom Blonde	My radiation technician
Dr. F	My plastic surgeon
Dr. S	My wound specialist
Dr. D	My bone specialist

ABOUT THE AUTHOR

Jamie Batson currently teaches high school and Adult Education in Texas. She has five teaching certifications, has taught in every grade level, all core subjects, and many elective courses. She is currently teaching all high school core subjects in a resource style special education setting, and teaching writing part time through a local Junior College Adult Education Division some nights. She has a wonderful husband who has put up with her for nearly 24 years, and counts her blessings daily.

You may contact her through email at jcbatson@hotmail.com.